Health Informatics

(formerly Computers in Health Care)

Kathryn J. Hannah   Marion J. Ball
Series Editors

D1264376

Health Informatics Series
(formerly Computers in Health Care)

Series Editors
Kathryn J. Hannah   Marion J. Ball

Dental Informatics
Integrating Technology into the Dental Environment
L.M. Abbey and J. Zimmerman

Health Informatics Series
Evaluating the Organizational Impact of Healthcare Information Systems, Second Edition
J.G. Anderson and C.E. Aydin

Ethics and Information Technology
A Case-Based Approach to a Health Care System in Transition
J.G. Anderson and K.W. Goodman

Aspects of the Computer-Based Patient Record
M.J. Ball and M.F. Collen

Performance Improvement Through Information Management
Health Care's Bridge to Success
M.J. Ball and J.V. Douglas

Strategies and Technologies for Healthcare Information
Theory into Practice
M.J. Ball, J.V. Douglas, and D.E. Garets

Nursing Informatics
Where Caring and Technology Meet, Third Edition
M.J. Ball, K.J. Hannah, S.K. Newbold, and J.V. Douglas

Healthcare Information Management Systems
A Practical Guide, Second Edition
M.J. Ball, D.W. Simborg, J.W. Albright, and J.V. Douglas

Healthcare Information Management Systems
Cases, Strategies, and Solutions, Third Edition
M.J. Ball, C.A. Weaver, and J.M. Kiel

Clinical Decision Support Systems
Theory and Practice
E.S. Berner

Strategy and Architecture of Health Care Information Systems
M.K. Bourke

Information Networks for Community Health
P.F. Brennan, S.J. Schneider, and E. Tornquist

Informatics for the Clinical Laboratory
A Practical Guide for the Pathologist
D.F. Cowan

James M. Walker   Eric J. Bieber
Frank Richards
Editors

Implementing an Electronic Health Record System

With the Collaboration of Sandra A. Buckley

With 22 illustrations

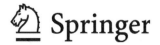 Springer

James M. Walker, MD
Chief Medical Information Officer
Geisinger Health System
Danville, PA, 17822, USA

Frank Richards
Chief Information Officer
Geisinger Health System
Danville, PA 17822, USA

Eric J. Bieber, MD
Senior Vice President
Chair of OB/GYN
Medical Director
Women's Service Line
Geisinger Health System
Danville, PA 17822, USA

Series Editors:
Kathryn J. Hannah, PhD, RN
Adjunct Professor, Department of
    Community Health Science
Faculty of Medicine
The University of Calgary
Calgary, Alberta T2N 4N1, Canada

Marion J. Ball EdD
Vice President, Clinical Solutions
2 Hamill Road
Quadrangle 359 West
Healthlink, Inc.
Baltimore, MD 21210
and
Adjunct Professor
The Johns Hopkins University
School of Nursing
Baltimore, MD 21205, USA

British Library Cataloging-in-Publication Data
A catalogue record for this book is available from the British Library

Library of Congress Control Number: 1846283302

First published 2005 in hardcover as ISBN 1-85233-826-1

ISBN 10: 1-84628-330-2   eISBN 1-84628-115-6
ISBN 13: 978-1-84628-330-7

Printed on acid-free paper.

Printed in the United States of America.   (SPI/EB)

9 8 7 6 5 4 3 2 1

springer.com

Series Preface

This series is directed to healthcare professionals who are leading the transformation of health care by using information and knowledge to advance the quality of patient care. Launched in 1988 as Computers in Health Care, the series offers a broad range of titles: some are addressed to specific professions such as nursing, medicine, and health administration; others to special areas of practice such as trauma and radiology. Still other books in the series focus on interdisciplinary issues, such as the computer-based patient record, electronic health records, and networked healthcare systems.

Renamed Health Informatics in 1998 to reflect the rapid evolution in the discipline now known as health informatics, the series continues to add titles that contribute to the evolution of the field. In the series, eminent experts, serving as editors or authors, offer their accounts of innovation in health informatics. Increasingly, these accounts go beyond hardware and software to address the role of information in influencing the transformation of healthcare delivery systems around the world. The series also increasingly focuses on "peopleware" and the organizational, behavioral, and societal changes that accompany the diffusion of information technology in health services environments.

These changes will shape health services in the new millennium. By making full and creative use of the technology to tame data and to transform information, health informatics will foster the development of the knowledge age in health care. As coeditors, we pledge to support our professional colleagues and the series readers as they share the advances in the emerging and exciting field of health informatics.

Kathryn J. Hannah
Marion J. Ball

Preface

Implementing an electronic health record system (EHR) that includes computerized physician order entry (CPOE) has gone from being a dream of researchers and visionaries to becoming a business necessity (1).

Two highly visible forces have driven this change. The first is public awareness of dismayingly high rates of avoidable errors in healthcare (2–6). The second is the demonstration that CPOE can reduce medical errors and costs significantly (7–9). In the most careful study to-date, the Center for Information Technology Leadership estimates that the adoption of high-performance ambulatory computerized physician order entry could save a total of $44 billion each year in healthcare costs (10).

Additional forces, less visible, but nonetheless important, strengthen the case for EHRs: Wennberg and others have documented wide, unexplained variations in the processes and outcomes of care—coupled with the frequently documented relationship between variation and poor quality (11–16). Expensive, inefficient, paper-based information management processes have become unacceptable in the face of internal performance improvement and external regulatory reporting needs that are increasing steadily in complexity and scope.

The forces encouraging the adoption of EHRs with CPOE have been brought to focus by the inclusion of CPOE as one of the core measures of quality care by coalitions of employers, most notably the Leapfrog Group (composed of more than 140 public and private organizations that provide healthcare benefits for 25 million people—www.leapfroggroup.org). Payers, including the Center for Medicare and Medicaid Services, have added their clout (9, 17–23).

Despite the powerful forces now driving adoption of EHRs, many care delivery organizations (CDOs—defined as any organization, large or small, that performs patient diagnosis and treatment), along with the majority of independent physician practices, continue to find challenges in implementing a high-performance EHR (one that includes CPOE).

What Constitutes an EHR?

At a high level, increasing patient safety, improving the quality and precision of care, and increasing the efficiency of clinical and administrative processes are compelling reasons to implement an EHR. To achieve these goals, the core functions of test results display, order entry, clinical messaging, and documentation of clinical observations and plans must be included in the EHR.

Many additional processes either need to be incorporated into the EHR, or supported effectively by it, for an implementation to achieve optimal results. As Mark Frisse, the healthcare informatics researcher and consultant, highlights with his healthcare information value chain (24), an EHR should be part of an information system that includes:

- Scheduling and demand management
- Determination of patient eligibility
- Referrals and authorizations
- Information access and reporting
- Care management
- Claims submissions
- Practice management, premium billing, capitation/risk pools, claims processing
- Health risk appraisals and wellness education
- Secure e-mail

While the focus of this book is on implementing an EHR that performs the core functions, your organization will need to think about which of these additional functions need to be included to achieve your business goals.

Constraints

The costs of implementing an EHR are substantial. By the time high-speed, fault tolerant networks, servers, personal computers (PCs), and other hardware are added to software costs and the salaries needed for a capable information technology (IT) team, the total will be measured in the millions of dollars annually, even for healthcare organizations employing only 100 physicians. In addition, the contributions of clinicians' and managers' that are needed for system design, user training and non-IT operational support will represent a significant new set of demands on organizational (especially managerial) attention and energy. This comes at a time when cost reduction and quality improvement requirements have already imposed more change on many CDOs and independent physician practices than they have resources to cope with effectively. Finally, despite studies suggesting that EHRs have the potential to save society and money (25), not a single persuasive case study has demonstrated overall savings.

The few careful studies of the quality effects of EHRs have been performed on isolated components of custom-built EHRs that are supported by research oriented IT teams. These efficacy studies demonstrate what can be accomplished under optimal conditions. But we do not know whether these findings can be extended to organizations that use commercial software, that are supported by internal IT teams who must focus on the practical issues of implementation and support, and whose clinicians are less familiar with EHRs. Nor do we know whether (or how) clinical decision support (CDS) can effectively address the hundreds of decision rules that would be required to improve provision of basic healthcare (6).

Commercially available (and custom developed) EHRs are still relatively immature. Usability remains sub-optimal, discouraging clinician adoption and making efficiency benefits difficult to realize (26–28). Substantial local customization is difficult, but always required. Because we are early in the evolution of EHRs, few products have even a small group of genuinely successful implementations (defined as in use by all clinicians for results viewing, clinical messaging, order entry and documentation).

The organization's existing legacy software systems will require interfacing with the EHR. These interfaces will represent substantial ongoing costs that most organizations will not be able to avoid in the near or mid-term.

Because of the inherent complexity of healthcare information needs and EHR software, it is rare for anyone working either for the vendor or the CDO to understand the product comprehensively. CDOs and vendors alike have difficulty training and retaining people with the technical and organizational change skills to manage implementations. Neither competencies nor training are standardized. Physician champions and clinician domain experts (see Glossary) make crucial contributions to implementations, but few come to the project with a realistic understanding of information systems or of the organizational changes needed to implement a system that addresses all of the organization's core processes.

Our Experience

This book arises out of our organization's experience with implementing an integrated outpatient and inpatient EHR across an integrated healthcare system. Since its founding in 1915, Geisinger has served a 31-county, largely rural area of northeastern and central Pennsylvania. Our 600 primary care and specialist physicians see approximately 1.5 million outpatient visits a year in 43 outpatient practice sites. In one of our hospitals, Geisinger Medical Center, 280 employed physicians and 200 residents and fellows provide tertiary and quaternary care for a large region of Pennsylvania. Our community hospital, Geisinger Wyoming Valley, has an open staff model and few residents or fellows. Discharges from Geisinger's inpatient units total over 29,000 annually. Our health maintenance organization, Geisinger Health Plan, covers approximately 243,000 patient lives. Our active EHR database included 2.4 million patients as of December 2003.

Our experience has included early failures based squarely on what were at the time widely-accepted best practices (see Chapter 14). We have also benefited from many of the critical success factors for implementing an EHR (29). Among them: unwavering senior leadership commitment; a visible and effective EHR physician champion; a collegial approach to decision making; widespread involvement and support of physicians; project management, financial and technical resources; and a high-quality product provided by a stable vendor. The implementation has ranged from primary care practices in geographically isolated rural communities to hospital-based subspecialty practices and a quaternary-care hospital. Recently, we have extended EHR access to 14,000 patients throughout our practice sites and to several hundred affiliated physicians. Given the heterogeneity of our own system, we believe that our experience in implementing an EHR has wide applicability to small, medium and large groups and CDOs.

Goals of the Book

Our implementation team receives increasing numbers of requests for site visits and other forms of consultation on implementing an EHR. While we enjoy these opportunities to share what we have learned, we are invariably frustrated by time constraints. This book is our effort to package a combined site visit and consulting engagement into a convenient form.

Our goal is to provide a practical handbook that will help you address the strategic and tactical challenges of implementing an EHR successfully. It combines research-based principles, industry best practices and our own experience. For many implementation issues there are several possible approaches and no well-tested best practice. We have used different approaches at different times and places during our implementation. The book aims to represent this multiplicity and to present the pros and cons of each approach rather than reducing our experience to deceptively simple answers. Although we have planned and edited the book to be read through as a comprehensive guide, the individual chapters are also designed to stand on their own as discussions of specific topics.

Audience

This book has been designed for EHR project team managers and directors, implementation teams, clinician champions of EHR implementations, other clinician informaticians, Chief Medical Information Officers, Chief Information Officers, consultants, EHR vendors and students of healthcare informatics. Chief Medical Officers, Chief Operating Officers and Chief Executive Officers may also find it useful. We have assumed familiarity with the basics of the Western healthcare systems, health care informatics, and project management. (Please see Glossary for any unfamiliar terms. To find definitions for terms we have not included, go to www.google.com and enter the term plus the word "definition", e.g. "project management definition".)

We are indebted to many beyond our organization for helpful insights. Mark Frisse has been particularly generous with his time and insights. We look forward to your questions and comments. Please send them to jmwalker@communityERH.com.

James M. Walker, MD
Eric J. Bieber, MD
Frank Richards

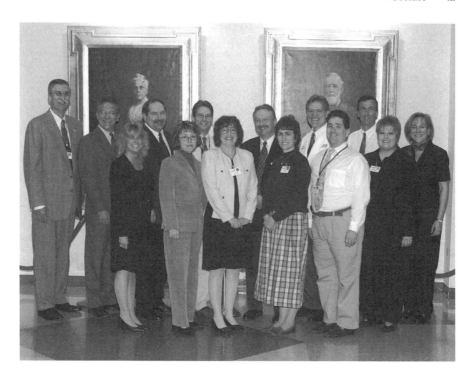

References

1. iHealthBeat. CPOE, EMRs top IT executives' projects. In; 2003.
2. Kohn L, Corrigan J, Donaldson M, editors. To Err Is Human: Building a Safer Health System. Washington, D.C.: NATIONAL ACADEMY PRESS; 1999.
3. Davis K, Schoenbaum SC, Collins KS. Room for Improvement: Patients Report on the Quality of Their Health Care. In; 2002.
4. Barker KN, Flynn EA, Pepper GA, Bates DW. Medication Errors Observed in 36 Health Care Facilities. Arch Intern Med 2002;162:1897.
5. iHealthBeat. IOM report: IT 'critical element' for health system reform. In; 2002.
6. McGlynn EA, Asch SM, Adams J. The Quality of Health Care Delivered to Adults in the United States. NEJM 2003;348:2635–2645.
7. Bates D, Cohen M, Leape L, Overhage J, Shabot M. Reducing the Frequency of Errors in Medicine Using Information Technology. JAMIA 2001;8:299.
8. iHealthBeat. North Carolina hospital scores with CPOE. In; 2003.
9. Midwest Business Group on Health. Reducing the Cost of Poor-Quality Health Care through Responsible Purchasing Leadership. In: Midwest Business Group on Health in collaboration with Juran Institute, Inc. and The Severyn Group, Inc.; 2003.
10. Johnston D, Pan E, Middleton B. Finding the Value in Healthcare Information Technologies. In. Boston MA: Center for IT Leadership, Partners HealthCare; 2002.
11. Wennberg J. Are hospital services rationed in New Haven or over-utilized in Boston? Lancet 1987;1(1185).
12. Wennberg J. The paradox of appropriate care. JAMA 1987;258:2568.
13. Wennberg J. The association between local diagnostic testing intensity and subsequent invasive cardiac procedures. JAMA 1996;275:1161.

14. Wennberg D. Variation in Carotid Endarterectomy Mortality in the Medicare Population: Trial Hospitals, Volume, and Patient Characteristics. JAMA 1998;279:1278.

15. Leape L, Park R, Solomon D. Relation between surgeons' practice volumes and geographic variation in the rate of carotid endarterectomy. NEJM 1989;321:653–657.

16. Wise P, Eisenberg L. What do regional variations in the rates of hospitalization of children really mean? NEJM 1989;320:1209.

17. Karash J. Official predicts boom in health-care information technology. Star 2002 Oct. 22, 2002.

18. CMS. CMS Issues Final Quality-Assesment and Performance-Improvement Conditions of Participation for Hospitals. In: CMS; 2003.

19. Kowalczyk L. For doctors, bonuses for quality care. Globe Staff 2002 02.11.07.

20. iHealthBeat. Employer group to offer physician bonuses for IT use. In; 2003.

21. iHealthBeat. Wisconsin bill would pay hospitals for IT use. In; 2003.

22. iHealthBeat. American Heart Association says IT use could curb medical errors. In; 2002.

23. iHealthBeat. California health plan will tie hospital coverage to quality efforts. In; 2002.

24. Frisse MC. The business value of health care information technology. JAMIA 1999;6:361.

25. Johnston D, Pan E, Walker J. The Value of Computerized Provider Order Entry in Ambulatory Settings. Boston: Center for Information Technology Leadership; 2003.

26. Ornstein C. Hospital Heeds Doctors, Suspends Use of Software. Times 2003 03.01.22.

27. Teich J. What is wrong with the electronic medical record? In: AMIA Fall Conference; 1999 11-9-99; Washington, DC: AMIA; 1999.

28. Zhang. Usability Problems with electronic medical record. In: AMIA Fall Conference; 1999 11-9-99; Washington, DC: AMIA; 1999.

29. Ash JS, Stavri PZ, Kuperman GJ. A Consensus Statement on Considerations for a Successful CPOE Implementation. JAMIA 10:229–234 (2003) 2003.

Acknowledgments

Like a successful EHR implementation, this book represents the combined efforts of a large and skilled team. The authors and editors have taken time from demanding implementation and production-support responsibilities to reflect on the principles and methods they have learned over ten years of planning, implementing, and assessing EHR-related projects. We are all in their debt.

Tom Abendroth and Mark Frisse provided invaluable advice. Deserée Karns' skill and hard work and humor kept the project (and me) on time and on target. Shirley, Peter, Katie, and my patients remind me of the reasons we are building EHRs.

Finally, this book is dedicated to Glenn Steele, without whose vision and support it would not have been written.

James M. Walker, MD

Contents

Part III   IMPLEMENTATION

Part IV   SUMMARY AND PROSPECT

Contributors

Jean A. Adams, RN
Director, Information Technology, Geisinger Health System, Danville, PA

Diane L. Barnes
Lead Systems Analyst, Information Technology, Geisinger Health System, Danville, PA

Eric J. Bieber, MD
Senior Vice President, Chair of OB/GYN; Medical Director, Women's Service Line Geisinger Health System, Danville, PA

Joseph E. Bisordi, MD
Associate Chief Medical Officer, Geisinger Health System, Danville, PA

Elizabeth A. Boyer
Program Director, Information Technology, Geisinger Health System, Danville, PA

Sandra A. Buckley
Director, Editorial Office, Geisinger Health System, Danville, PA

Janet S. Byron, MPH
Lead Systems Analyst, Information Technology, Geisinger Health System, Danville, PA

Linda M. Culp
Program Director, Information Technology, Geisinger Health System, Danville, PA

Kathleen M. Dean
Associate Vice President, System Marketing, Geisinger Health System, Danville, PA

W. Todd Gibson, MHA
Director, Revenue Cycle Operations, Geisinger Health System, Danville, PA

Roy A. Gill, MD
Senior Medical Informatician, Geisinger Health System, Danville, PA

BRUCE H. HAMORY, MD
Executive Vice President and Chief Medical Officer, Geisinger Health System, Danville, PA

ELLIE E. HENRY
Manager of Center for Best Practices, Geisinger Health System, Danville, PA

MICHAEL J. KOMAR, MD
Director, Gastroenterology, Geisinger Health System, Danville, PA

WANDA L. KRUM
Lead Systems Analyst, Information Technology, Geisinger Health System, Danville, PA

MICHAEL C. LAMPMAN
Senior Systems Analyst, Information Technology, Geisinger Health System, Danville, PA

JACK D. LATSHAW, MAEd
Assistant Director, Technology Education Services, Geisinger Health System, Danville, PA

FRANK RICHARDS
Chief Information Officer, Geisinger Health System, Danville, PA

KIMBERLY A. ROKITA, MSRD
Program Director, Information Technology, Geisinger Health System, Danville, PA

MICHAEL W. SOBACK
Director II, Information Technology, Geisinger Health System, Danville, PA

STEPHEN T. TINGLEY, BO
University Physician, Urgent Care, University Health Services, The Pennsylvania State University, University Park, PA

JOAN E. TOPPER
Director, eHealth & Performance Improvement, Geisinger Health System, Danville, PA

JAMES M. WALKER, MD
Chief Medical Information Officer, Geisinger Health System, Danville, PA

TRACEY W. WOLF, MHA
Associate Vice President, Academic Affairs and Center for Health Research & Rural Advocacy, Geisinger Health System, Danville, PA

DAVID L. YOUNG
Program Director, Information Technology, Web Services, Geisinger Health System, Danville, PA

EDWARD J. ZYCH, ESQUIRE
Senior Managing Litigation Counsel, Geisinger Health System, Danville, PA

Part One
Preparation

1
Organizational Climate

SANDRA A. BUCKLEY, JOSEPH E. BISORDI, and BRUCE H. HAMORY

Introduction

Many factors influence the organizational structure of care delivery organizations (CDOs). These include location (urban vs. rural), organizational mission, size, complexity of services offered (primary and specialty care), and availability of sufficient funds to support operations and capital investments. CDOs that are part of a university are even more complex, with added administrative staff required for their teaching and research missions.

Before the 1990s, Geisinger's information technology (IT) investments were lagging behind those of non-healthcare organizations. This was almost universally true for CDOs, which, as late as 2002, were still spending only 3% of gross revenue on IT. (Other information-driven businesses, such as banks, were spending 9%.) Other industries demonstrated early on that IT investments could enable them to extract more value from their investments over time. American Airlines' Sabre® reservation system makes it easy to determine flight availability and book a flight. Federal Express implemented a tracking system that reduced delays and increased customer satisfaction. Toyota reduced the maximum time any part was present in an assembly plant to two hours.

Healthcare's initial investment in IT was largely driven by reimbursement issues and the need to report and track finances. Billing, business, and accounting systems were implemented before clinical systems.

In the early 1990s, Geisinger embarked on a program to enhance clinic practice by providing an integrated system of care serving the population of a large, mostly rural 31-county area. It became clear that to do this successfully would require radical change, including a quantum leap in information management. In 1995, the Board of Directors approved a multi-year IT strategic plan that included major investments to acquire and implement an electronic health record (EHR) system. This decision was based on many factors, including the need to improve communication of clinical data across the integrated delivery system, improve patient safety (through point-of-care clinical decision support), reduce practice variability, introduce best practices, reduce costs, increase revenues, and meet regulatory requirements efficiently. As the EHR was implemented, it became apparent that Geisinger could leverage these IT investments—not feasible elsewhere within our market—to increase cooperation with patients and referring physicians.

Today, Geisinger is a national leader in the use of healthcare information technology. In 1999, and again in 2002, Geisinger was named one of the country's "Most Wired" healthcare companies, serving as a national model for healthcare IT. In 2001, Geisinger was the only healthcare organization to be selected as a finalist in the Wharton Infosys Awards for applying IT to business transformation. In 2003, the Chief Information Officer (CIO), Frank Richards, was named one of the 100 leaders of American information technology.

This chapter will describe how we benefited from and transformed our organizational climate to make maximum use of healthcare information technology.

Geisinger Health System Overview

We have benefited from a number of factors that have supported information technology innovation. Key factors include:

- Knowledgeable, visionary leaders
- Location
- A collegial, service-oriented culture
- Physician leadership
- A strong financial base
- A salaried physician practice
- The confluence of business needs and technology developments

Mission

Geisinger's mission is to enhance the region's quality of life through an integrated health service organization based on a balanced program of patient care, education, research, and community service. In 1915, Abigail A. Geisinger founded the George F. Geisinger Memorial Hospital in Danville, PA (current population approximately 6,500). The hospital was designed from the onset as a comprehensive facility that would offer specialized medical care to people in rural central and northeastern Pennsylvania. Geisinger's culture is inspired by the legacy of Abigail Geisinger. She challenged the first Surgeon-in-Chief, Dr. Harold Leighton Foss, to: "make my hospital right; make it the best." Throughout the years, the Geisinger community has remained faithful to this vision, perhaps best expressed as: "We can make it here; we can make it right; we can make it the best".

The Geisinger Health System includes the Geisinger Clinic, a multispecialty physician group practice that employs more than 600 salaried physicians and operates the largest ambulatory care program in Pennsylvania, including 42 widely distributed primary-care practices. Geisinger facilities also include Geisinger Medical Center, a large tertiary care teaching hospital with 450-licensed beds; Geisinger Wyoming Valley, a 200-bed community hospital; Marworth, a 77-bed drug and alcohol rehabilitation center; and an ambulatory surgery center. Geisinger Medical Center maintains an active Level I Regional Trauma Center supported by "Life Flight®," a three-helicopter air ambulance service. In fiscal year 2002 (July 1, 2001 through June 30, 2002), Geisinger recorded more than 1.5 million outpatient visits and 30,000 discharges from its inpatient units. Our primary care practices serve about 500,000 patients annually. Geisinger Health Plan, created in 1972 and restructured and incorporated in 1985, has become one of the nation's largest rural health maintenance organization (HMO).

Leadership History

Geisinger's physician leadership has been remarkably visionary. Its first President and CEO, Dr. Harold Foss, was a surgeon who joined the Mayo Clinic in 1913 as a fellow in surgery. Dr. Foss, a pioneer in rural healthcare administration, led the George F. Geisinger Memorial Hospital (later the Geisinger Medical Center) through its first 44 years, replicating the multi-disciplinary clinic/hospital model he learned at the Mayo Clinic. In 1958, Dr. Foss was succeeded by Leonard Bush, MD, an orthopedic surgeon, who served as President and CEO through 1974.

Dr. Bush was succeeded by Henry Hood, MD, a neurosurgeon who served from 1974 to 1990. Having earned an undergraduate degree in hotel management before his medical degree, Dr. Hood brought a unique business perspective to Geisinger. Under Dr. Hood's leadership Geisinger accepted the challenge of state healthcare planners to use the tertiary-care capabilities of GMC to meet the healthcare needs of the entire region. Dr. Hood led a major expansion of the Medical Center, which doubled in size between 1978 and 1981 with the acquisition and development of our primary-care practices. The Marworth Alcohol & Chemical Dependency Treatment Center and the Geisinger Wyoming Valley Medical Center were also acquired (or built) during this period. The Geisinger Medical Management Corporation began providing management consulting and other medical services (home care, infusion therapy, retail pharmacies) to CDOs, both inside and outside the system.

As this large, geographically dispersed healthcare system developed, it became apparent that consistent business processes (administrative and clinical) were needed to unite the many parts into an effective whole. Dr. Hood recognized that a standardized IT infrastructure and software applications would make these goals feasible. Under his leadership Geisinger investigated EHRs, but concluded that the technology was too immature to be useful.

Stuart Heydt, MD, an oral surgeon, succeeded Dr. Hood in 1990. In the early 1990s, a team led by the COO (Frank Trembulak) and the CIO (Pat Thompson), recommended centralizing IT operations and building the IT infrastructure required to support a high-performance ambulatory EHR (see Chapter 4). With the addition of Joseph Bisordi, MD (Chair of Nephrology) as Senior Vice President for Medical Informatics, this team led the ambulatory EHR implementation, which reached all 42 clinic sites and 600 physicians. Also during this period, Geisinger's Radiology Department implemented an electronic digital image storage and distribution system, making most radiology images available on PCs throughout the organization.

In 2000, with the outpatient EHR implementation well underway, we began a second round of strategic planning to identify ways to leverage our investments in the EHR. Recognizing the value of the EHR to Geisinger clinicians, we decided to find ways for patients and independent regional physicians to access the EHR also. (For details, see Chapters 19 and 20.) In 2003, we extended this information to include hospitals outside the Geisinger system.

Today, Geisinger's fifth President and CEO is Glenn Steele, Jr., MD, PhD, a nationally known surgical oncologist and healthcare leader. Under his leadership, Geisinger is extending its clinical information systems and expertise to the region and the nation. Geisinger's Center for Health Research & Rural Advocacy, under the leadership of Walter "Buzz" Stewart, PhD, has established itself as one of the nation's premier sites for rigorous real-world research on the effectiveness of EHRs to improve healthcare quality and efficiency.

Organizational Structure

The committed, visionary leadership of Geisinger's Board of Directors has been instrumental in moving Geisinger's strategic initiatives forward over decades. Its members have a strong commitment to the local community and to Geisinger's excellence. They have consistently provided the resources needed to carry out strategic program planning, including investments in IT. The shared commitment and vision of the Board and the executive management team, sustained over time, may have been the single most important factor in Geisinger's success in implementing an EHR.

Location, Location, Location

Geisinger is headquartered in the small town of Danville, PA. Our largely rural service area extends over 20,000 square miles. This geographic isolation created a need for innovative methods of linking the system together, to make it more than just the sum of its disparate parts.

Culture

Geisinger has had, since its beginning, a community focus. Our original model for care was based on a physically contiguous multi-disciplinary group practice. This coordinated, collaborative model of care depends critically on the ability to share information (originally in the form of a shared paper chart). As the organization expanded, we needed to replicate the benefits of this model across an expanded geographical footprint.

Our population base (2.3 million) is very stable. Many of our patients live in a house that has been passed down from generation to generation. This is also true of our employees, who are strongly committed to the region. Recruiting from outside the local area is more difficult than in urban environments. However, the stability of our employee base has a positive effect on our ability to retain good employees. The average turnover rate in our IT Department is 5%–half the national average. The average length of service is approximately 11 years. Many of the current leaders in the IT department (including the CIO) started their careers in other Geisinger departments (pharmacy, nursing, dietary, laboratory, and management engineering). This diverse clinical background results in experienced, operationally sensitive IT teams and leaders.

Physician-Led

Geisinger's tradition of physician leadership ensures continued attention to the day-to-day realities of a busy clinical environment. All levels of the organization, from each practice to the executive suite have physician leaders, most of whom remain clinically active. The tradition of partnering physician and administrative leaders is replicated in IT. The Chief Medical Information Officer (CMIO), James M. Walker, MD, is partnered with the CIO, Frank Richards.

Financial Base

As a not-for-profit organization, Geisinger retains its earnings for investment in program improvements. With a strong balance sheet, Geisinger has had the financial strength and institutional patience to make the long-term investment in IT that an effective EHR requires. However, we began to realize significant returns on investment only after several years of financial investment. For example, paper chart pulls can only be eliminated when all clinicians use the EHR. Initially, the EHR is relatively empty of patient information; only after substantial information is put into it does the EHR become really valuable to clinicians. EHR software and implementation methodologies have improved markedly, but organizations considering an EHR must be aware that both hard work and patience will be needed before the full benefits of the project are realized.

Salaried Physicians

Geisinger physicians are salaried. Compensation includes a base salary and a variable bonus based on achievement of specific incentive criteria. These criteria are aligned with system goals, such as patient satisfaction, clinical performance, and financial performance. This incentive system has provided valuable motivation for physician adoption of the EHR.

In addition to our salaried physicians, about 150 non-Geisinger physicians care for patients at our community hospital. For these physicians, the primary incentive for EHR use is improved efficiency and care quality. They value easy access to clinical information (e.g., test results, radiology images, outpatient notes, and procedure notes). They also value the convenience of e-messaging that is linked to the patient's record. Finally, HIPAA-compliant access to the EHR in their offices and homes gives physicians gratifying new flexibility in the way they work. These benefits create increasing demand for more access and for the ability to enter notes and orders into the system remotely.

Confluence of Business Needs and Technology Development

Fortunately, Geisinger's increasing need for business and clinical information systems coincided with the maturation of information technology that could meet those needs. In the late 1980s, we deferred initial consideration of a system-wide EHR because it was clear that the available technology was inadequate to meet the challenge. Only a few years later, a number of technologies (E-mail, Web technologies, core EHRs, digital imaging) had matured sufficiently to make an EHR attractive and feasible. While these emerging technologies were becoming available, a number of factors prevented most CDOs from implementing an EHR. Prominent among these were the managerial and intellectual fragmentation of most organizations at that time, immature implementation methodologies, and the number and complexity of business processes that an EHR must support.

Communications

Effective communication is frequent, accurate, succinct, tailored to the needs of the audience(s), delivered by trusted messengers, and accompanied by opportunities for feedback (1). Particularly in the case of an EHR—which will inevitably change work roles, access to information, and monitoring of individual and group performance—a comprehensive communication plan is essential to maintain your organization's focus and motivation.

Once the executive leadership and Board of Directors agreed to proceed with implementation of an EHR, we began to develop a plan for communicating the decision to the organization. The physician champion (the Senior Vice President for Medical Informatics) created a specific, consistent message that was presented at all levels of the organization. The message emphasized the importance of efficient information management in clinical care and the inclusiveness of the strategic planning process.

The message focused on five primary objectives for the EHR project: improving access (with system-wide scheduling); reducing costs; enhancing clinical communications; improving business processes; and providing clinical decision support. It included projected EHR benefits in each of these dimensions. The presentation concluded with a scenario-based patient encounter that took a patient from the initial phone call for an appointment through check out following the office visit. Other scenarios were also demonstrated, including patient telephone calls, electronic results review, and messaging among clinical staff. The implementation timeline was explained. The project remained as an agenda item on all organizational meetings with regular progress reports, emphasizing leadership's commitment to its success.

The physician champion gave these presentations to physicians at all levels and locations within the organization. This assured that physicians' questions and concerns could be understood. It also helped emphasize that the organization and its physician leadership were committed to the extensive change entailed by this project. Physicians who had already implemented the EHR were encouraged to describe their experience in organizational meetings to create a shared sense of progress and success.

A similar process of formal presentations was employed several years later to communicate the subsequent e-Health strategy and the inpatient EHR implementation.

Summary

An institution contemplating an EHR must have buy-in from the very top of the organization (including its board) and be willing to make information technology part of the organization's strategic plan. Resources for initial and ongoing IT investments must be committed—and the institution must have the patience to wait for the returns on those investments.

EHR implementation is not easy, but it can transform your organization. Change on this scale creates the opportunity to rethink work processes, often resulting in more efficient operations. The EHR provides administrators and clinicians a powerful tool for institutionalizing process improvements. In fact, we have found that the EHR attracts clinicians and managers with a passion for quality improvement. Identify, hire, train and promote these people. Their leadership will be one of the primary benefits of the EHR project—and one of the critical factors for its ongoing success.

Additional Reading

Kotter J. *Leading Change.* Boston: Harvard Business School Press; 1996.
Although not directed specifically to healthcare, Kotter's book outlines a comprehensive approach to creating an organizational climate in which change is likely to succeed.

2
Needs Assessment

Jean A. Adams and Linda M. Culp

Implementing an EHR requires that you conduct a needs assessment, identify and quantify measures of success, and determine the methods for maximizing ongoing benefit realization. This chapter will address each of these needs.

What Is the Definition of a Needs Assessment?

We define needs assessment as a systematic process to develop an accurate understanding of the strengths and weaknesses of a business process in terms of efficiency and quality. This understanding is used to set and prioritize goals, to develop a plan, and to allocate resources. A formal needs assessment requires that you understand:

1. The goals of the proposed project
2. The current processes and workflows
3. The gap between #1 and #2 (above)—the gap analysis
4. The capabilities and limitations of the software in addressing this gap
5. The associated risks (technical and operational)

Why a Needs Assessment?

A needs assessment defines a department's priorities and lays out an organized approach for allocating resources. In addition, it helps to avoid many pitfalls, including:

- Missing stakeholder needs
- "Scope creep"—the gradual increase of the number of project deliverables
- Missed deadlines
- Unmet project goals
- Budget over-runs

To maximize the benefits realized, the EHR needs assessment should be completed prior to purchasing the EHR software or making process changes.

Strategic Goals

In the initial stages of considering an EHR, we agreed on five high-level goals:

1. Enhance clinical communication (especially primary care provider communication).
2. Obtain structured data for quality improvement and practice analysis.

3. Provide access to patient information.
4. Enable clinical decision support.
5. Produce financial benefits (cost savings, as well as revenue enhancements).
6. Today, we would add a sixth goal - Increase process efficiency. Accomplishing this goal is critical to improving care quality as well as business viability. It is also critical to motivating active EHR use by clinicians and patients, without which none of the other goals will be achieved.

Next, we created seven high-level vision teams composed of senior managers, physicians, IT personnel, and patients, whose task was to think strategically about the organization's goals of delivering healthcare efficiently to a rural population.

The teams prioritized the EHR needs regarding:

• Order management
• Results display (radiology, laboratory, and pathology)
• Patient scheduling
• Registration and checkout referral management
• Utilization management
• Information security

The teams developed high-level proposals for core processes based on industry best practices. They worked to an aggressive timeline (Table 2.1) to complete their final reports, which were then presented to the Board of Directors.

The teams were instructed not to restrict their design to fit the functionality limitations of existing software systems. Appendix 1 provides a high-level overview of the Vision teams' results.

After Board approval, we formed design teams to assess current workflows and design optimized workflows. They then assessed software functionality that would be needed to achieve the optimized workflows.

The core question we ask when conducting needs assessments is, Who needs what information, at what times, and in what locations, for what purposes? This question is asked for existing workflow processes and then reviewed when designing optimized workflows.

Needs assessment begins with a detailed walk-through of a practice site with the practice's primary stakeholders (managers, clinicians, and administrative staff). This walk-through is followed by a group meeting to determine a high-level understanding of the practice's needs. This provides the basis for detailed questions in subsequent group meetings. The follow-up meetings include a team of managers, physician leaders, nurses and clinical technicians. The initial meeting is two hours in length (we have found that shorter meetings are not as productive as longer ones, since part of every meeting involves reviewing issues addressed in prior meetings). An assigned interviewer documents the sessions; the full team reviews the documentation for accuracy and completeness. The team analyst (see Glossary) then converts the interviews into

TABLE 2.1. Vision Team Timelines.

Teams Identified and Formed	Weekly Team Meetings	Draft Report Review	Final Report and Presentation to Board
Month 0	Months 1 & 2	Month 3	Month 4

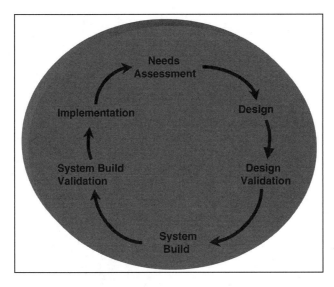

FIGURE 2.1. The role of a needs assessment in the implementation process.

process flow charts that are also reviewed by the team members. Appendix 2 is a sample of a completed "Needs Assessment."

It is often difficult for stakeholders to differentiate between a needs assessment and a wish list. Needs and wishes lie along a spectrum of utilization and feasibility. It is critical that the team understand (at the initial team meeting) the difference between the two. An item on a wish list might be attractive to the requestor, but have little impact on business quality or efficiency (or benefit only a few users). We record these requests as ideas for future development, but they naturally fall to the bottom of the priority list. In comparison, a need is critical to clinical or business operations and is relatively feasible. An example of a need would be a request that information be displayed in a consistent format that is usable for all users (See Figures 2.1 and 2.2).

Prioritizing Needs

As needs are identified in the needs assessment, they are rank-ordered into these categories:

- Required for initial implementation
- Required for Phase II
- Desirable, but not feasible
- Potentially counterproductive (the most frequent reason for this categorization is an item that would actually impede the work of some stakeholders)

To conduct interviews effectively, analysts need a positive attitude and the ability to listen patiently. Both of these traits were vital to facilitate the brainstorming phase of identifying needs. Once the analysts understand the workflows of the interviewees, they probe for needs that might otherwise be overlooked. The interviewer analyst employs a thorough, logical approach to analyzing workflows so that they can help the team identify all relevant needs.

Oscillation of a Request

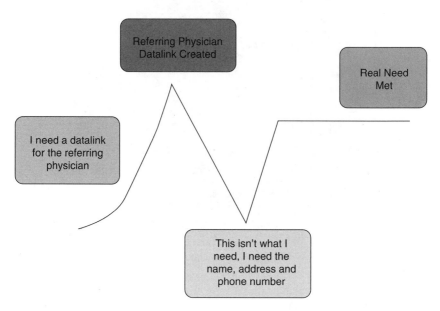

Referring Physician
Datalink Created

Real Need
Met

I need a datalink
for the referring
physician

This isn't what I
need, I need the
name, address and
phone number

FIGURE 2.2. If the implementation process is not followed, this figure represents the rework involved in understanding the needs of an end user.

After the team documents the needs assessment and documents the current work-flow and optimized workflow, the documents are shared with prospective EHR vendors. Vendors are given approximately two weeks to review this documentation. They are then invited to demonstrate at Geisinger their ability to meet the stated needs, using scenarios provided by the needs assessment team. Each software function demonstrated is identified as either currently available, planned, or out of the vendor's scope. This list is double-checked at the conclusion of the demonstration.

Depending on the scope of the project, vendor demonstrations may be divided into two sessions, conducted on the same day but by different teams. One team addresses operational needs; the other addresses technical needs. If these meetings are held separately, the two teams need to meet at the end of the day to develop a unified overview of the software's performance.

The next step is a point-by-point confirmation of the needs that the vendor's current product meets. This review forms the starting point for the gap analysis, the identification of which of the needs the vendor's product cannot meet. Appendix 3 provides an example of an initial gap analysis. The gap analysis also identifies workflows that need to be created, how the EHR software needs to be configured to support those workflows, the training needs, and vendor software development needs.

After stakeholders and the vendor verify the gap analysis, work sessions are conducted with operations personnel and the vendor to establish an action plan. These actions include a combination of:

- Vendor enhancements—Ensure that the enhancement agreements are included in the signed contract.

- Modified workflows to accommodate the remaining gaps
- Reprioritized needs—The process of needs assessment is iterative, with important needs continuing to surface at various stages of the process. Proposed additions are prioritized as above, with careful attention to avoiding scope creep.

Throughout this process, important goals need to be balanced. They include:

- Patient safety
- Healthcare quality
- Process efficiency
- Other organizational business plans and goals
- EHR usability

Measures of Success

After the gap analysis is completed, the next step is to identify measures of success. Widely agreed, explicit measures of success (short-term and long-term) are critical to the success of an implementation. They provide guidance to the implementation team and to the organization in making the myriad of decisions an implementation requires. They also provide the means of monitoring the progress of the project and communicating that progress. While predefined measures exert the most formative influence on an implementation, you will likely identify new measures as the implementation progresses (or modify existing measures based on ongoing review). For instance, we did not originally identify the reduction in manpower needs resulting from decreased chart pulls as a goal. However, by the sixth year of our outpatient implementation, we had eliminated 10 full-time positions in medical records and twelve full-time medical secretary positions in physician practices.

Success can be divided along two dimensions: care quality versus financial, and quantitative versus directional (Figure 2.3). Directional benefits (e.g., the ability to monitor prescribing patterns to identify suboptimal use of medicines) are difficult to quantify. On the other hand, the number of lines of transcription is a quantifiable measure. (We found that some outpatient clinics reduced their lines of transcription by 90% within a month of going live while other clinics increased dictation.)

Improved care processes can also be measured quantitatively. For example, the staff person who places a patient in the exam room is responsible for checking the patient's allergies and current medications. If prescription renewals are needed, they also enter

	Care Quality	Financial
Quantitative	Decrease time to first antibiotic in meningitis	Decrease chart pulls
Directional	FDA drug warnings	Patient Satisfaction

FIGURE 2.3. Success can be divided along two dimensions: care quality versus financial, and quantitative versus directional.

the medication order in the EHR for physician confirmation. In this case, the measure is the number of patients whose allergies and medications are reviewed (and documented) at each office visit. We established the baseline for this measure by reviewing paper charts. Post-implementation, we created a database that tallied the number of patients who had their allergy list and medication list reviewed at each visit for comparison.

To Measure or Not to Measure?

Early in the development phase of the outpatient EHR project, we decided not to identify and document measurements of success. The strategic importance of implementing an outpatient EHR was so compelling that the costs of measuring its effectiveness did not seem justified. We believed that many of the most important improvements the EHR enabled would be too pervasive to be measured accurately. Finally, we underestimated the critical value of explicit measures of success for guiding needed changes in the EHR (and its use by clinicians and managers) post-implementation. Based on this experience, we developed measures of success at the outset of our inpatient implementation and are using them to guide its development and evaluate its success.

Summary

Needs assessment is the foundation of a successful EHR implementation. It helps your organization to build consensus on goals for the project. It guides your choice of software vendor. It guides your design-build choices. It makes the project's successes and remaining opportunities apparent, guiding the evolution of your organization's EHR and your use of it.

Additional Reading

Witkin B, Altschuld J. *Planning and Conducting Needs Assessments: A Practical Guide.* Thousand Oaks, CA, Sage; 1995.
A readable, practical, comprehensive introduction.

3
Vendor Selection and Contract Negotiation

FRANK RICHARDS

Selecting an EHR vendor is like selecting your spouse. You expect the decision will be life-changing (you hope for the better) and that it will have a long-term effect. Also, you can be certain that if things don't work out, the separation will be painful.

Understanding your organization's business needs and its culture are essential to selecting not just the right software, but the right vendor partner as well. Misunderstandings over expected functionalities and delivery dates can quickly sour a business relationship.

Goal Definition

It was our goal to eventually have a single system that supported the entire spectrum of clinical care, particularly inpatient and outpatient. However, at the time we began planning in the early 1990s, no such system existed. We chose to implement ambulatory practices as our first priority, leaving the inpatient portion of the implementation for later. We did plan to incorporate data from existing systems, such as laboratory and radiology, into the EHR (regardless of whether the tests were ordered in the inpatient or outpatient setting). This became the first filter in the process of narrowing the field of potential software systems and vendors.

We prioritized our needs as follows:

- Provide access to existing clinical data (laboratory, pathology, radiology) using a single repository.
- Implement computerized physician order entry and clinical documentation in the ambulatory setting to enhance the referral process and incorporate clinical reminders and alerts.
- Implement an EHR in the hospitals that includes computerized physician order entry, clinical documentation and nursing documentation.

Because no single vendor had all the functionality required, we decided to concentrate on goals 1 and 2, and developed the objectives outlined in Chapter 2.

Defining Requirements

Because of the centrality of the EHR to our core businesses, we did not follow the usual process of defining requirements (i.e., issuing a request for proposal, system selection, and contracting). Since our core business is providing care, the path was more complex and needed to be closely aligned with Geisinger's overall business plan. The journey to define and select a system began in 1993 and took two and a half years to complete.

Throughout the early 1990s, our IT, Management Engineering, and Clinical and Administrative Management Departments engaged in a study of the state of technology as it might apply to a rural health system. This effort included redesigning work processes and visiting CDOs with EHRs in active use (Latter Day Saints Hospital, Salt Lake City, UT; Brigham and Women's Hospital, Boston, MA; BJC Health System, St. Louis, MO; and the Mayo Clinic, Rochester, MN). A small technical team was commissioned to develop a clinical data repository in partnership with a commercial software vendor. (Although that effort did not achieve its original goal, we learned a lot about the complexities of interface development.) All of these exercises helped us to create reasonable expectations and strengthened the working relationship among clinical and technical leaders.

The IT strategic plan, which was developed in concert with the organization's overall strategic plan and approved in May 1995, set out high-level objectives for the EHR project:

The Strategic intent is to function as a seamless organization serving as the region's health service leader. On behalf of those we serve, Geisinger Health System (GHS) will establish a delivery system designed to manage the continuum of care from healthy living through acute and chronic care. GHS will continually evaluate processes and implement improvements in health services, incorporating the most cost-effective utilization of resources to achieve measurable improvement in the health of our service area. GHS will strive to provide people throughout our service area with access to consistent quality in health care regardless of where they enter our system.

At that time, managed care was our primary business strategy and the EHR needed to support a managed care delivery system.

These corporate strategies led directly to IT priorities in four major areas: infrastructure, clinical systems, managed care, and business systems. Given the high demand for information systems, it was necessary to prioritize and sequence the work. A team of administrators, physicians and IT leaders were commissioned in 1995 to determine how the organization should invest its resources over a three-year period. The team developed four parameters on which to evaluate requests:

1. *Value*: The relationship of costs to benefits—an estimate of the direct quantifiable impact on the organization.
2. *Need*: What is the importance of the project to the multiple stakeholders? Is there strong sponsorship? Is there useable electronic information installed?
3. *Support of Geisinger's core strategy* to:
   • Increase the managed care membership of the health plan, our insurance company.
   • Reduce the cost of service.
   • Enhance customer access and satisfaction.
   • Integrate patient care across the organization.
   • Measure and improve the quality of care.
4. *Precedence*: Is the project required as a precursor to other critical projects?

Appendix 4 contains an example of the spreadsheet we used to document the rating that each potential project received in each of the four categories. They were coded from dark to light gray, making it easy to compare the relative strengths of the projects.

A set of primary and secondary objectives was identified using this methodology:

Primary

- Clinical data flow reengineering (to take advantage of automation)
- Physician productivity tools—Determine what computer-based tools physicians might find useful (medical reference material, presentation software, E-mail, and so on).
- Referral management—Streamline the referral management process from primary care to specialist.
- Ambulatory EHR—Focus first on an EHR in the outpatient areas, using technology to improve communications among care providers.
- Nurse triage—Provide a telephone nurse triage service supporting clinical pathways and documentation.
- Scheduling for all outpatient practices.

Secondary

- Point-of-service billing and collection.
- Transcription—Expand transcription services to all outpatient practices.
- Clinical data repository—Develop a repository for all clinical information, both inpatient and outpatient.
- Clinical Decision Support—Provide alerts and reminders at the point of care. Develop system-wide rules and guidelines.
- Teleradiology—Provide access to images for remote reading, eventually moving to all digital imaging.
- Clinical costing—Develop more robust models to analyze costs associated with care processes. Look for ways to improve quality and lower costs.

Other Needs

Other significant needs were deferred beyond the three-year horizon. These included support for inpatient clinical areas, outcomes analysis, expert systems, home access, and wellness programs. The plan summarized what the computerized patient record would accomplish for various constituencies:

Members/Patients

- Decreased waiting time
- No unnecessary repeated tests, interviews, or other data gathering
- Enhanced access to treatment
- More convenient communication with physician practices
- Consistent, best quality care across the health system

Clinicians

- Clinical information available in exam rooms, offices, and home
- Consistent care delivery across practices
- Actionable feedback on clinical performance
- Improved communication with colleagues
- Medical reference information available (electronic library)
- Extended geographic reach of specialist resources

Employers

- Documented improvement in employee health status
- Cost reductions
- Decreased pharmacy costs
- Better access to care

Software Selection

At this point, it was time to begin the formal process of vendor selection. A committee of eight physicians (mostly primary care) and IT leaders identified needs and surveyed the marketplace. They decided that the EHR software had to:

- Be in active clinic use
- Be scalable to more than 1,000,000 visits per year
- Support consolidated reporting for the entire organization
- Have a useable, easily learned interface.

(See Appendix 1 for the specific recommendations created by the seven design teams discussed in Chapter 2. These policies provided a detailed framework for EHR selection).

Results Reporting

The selection team eventually narrowed the field to two vendors through a series of trade shows, site visits and peer networking. Finally, we selected the EHR provided by the Epic Systems®, Inc. (Madison, WI). Factors for selecting Epic included the availability of a full range of products (scheduling, registration, EHR), its architecture (a single, scalable database), and the fact that it was currently in use by physicians in real-world clinic practices. Today's market offers an ever-widening selection of products installed at increasing numbers of sites. The size, type and culture of your organization will determine the system that's right for you.

After this rigorous process, our choice of vendor was based more on a high-level assessment of how their EHR could support optimized practices than on a detailed response to our request for a proposal regarding EHR functional capabilities. In retrospect, it was the right decision for us. Although specific software functions are important, the way those functions are integrated into large-scale work processes is critical. The overall fit of the system with your particular vision for processes and workflows cannot always be represented by the sum of individual functions. Scenario-based demonstrations that mimic your practice's workflows may give you a better feel for this overall fit.

Contract Negotiations

After completing the system selection, it is time to embark on contract negotiations (the marriage). Few IT contracts carry greater risk or have a greater potential for long-term positive impact than those for EHRs. Whereas most automated systems affect a single clinical or financial support service (e.g., billing, laboratory, radiology), EHRs directly affect all the core processes of healthcare. Once implemented successfully, such systems become an essential part of care processes and are very difficult to replace or to work without. In addition, your organization is installing an EHR in the expectation that it will be a long-term repository of healthcare information. You need a viable vendor who is interested in building a true partnership, where both parties are committed to the other's long-term success. It is also important that you have a plan and a contract in place to protect yourself in the event that the vendor can no longer support the system (the prenuptial agreement).

General approaches to contract negotiation are well documented (1). Some points related specifically to contracting for an EHR are worth noting. The specifics of any contract will be determined by the goals and situation of the CDO, but the risks inherent in an EHR system make the vendor relationship and the contract especially important. Consider some form of risk/reward sharing. Having the vendor at risk for a successful implementation will help to keep their attention during implementation, but beware of companies that give away too much. The long-term viability of your vendor is vital to your success. If a vendor sells its EHR and associated services too cheaply in order to gain clients, their long-term viability may be threatened.

Remember that there are no proven technologies for secure clinical data storage available or on the horizon. Unlike paper, which requires no special technology for access, electronic data in proprietary database structures may be difficult or impossible to retrieve without the vendor's programs. Make sure you have a plan for how you will access the data you are storing today or ten years in the future.

Some suggestions for inclusion in your contract:

Get the Source Code

Arrange for access to the source code. This may be by way of a contract provision that allows you to have a copy of the programs directly or an escrow agreement that entitles you to receive the latest version of the source code should the vendor be unable to support the software. You may not have the staff or the expertise that the vendor had, but having the source code will give you the option to fix bugs and keep the system running, even if you have to hire an outside firm to do the actual work.

Secure Your Data

Remember that the information in the system is one of your organization's most valuable assets. Include language in the contract that specifies how data conversion will be handled if the relationship is dissolved. If possible, you should have the ability to extract the data from the system without the vendor's assistance and put it into a standard format, so that it can be printed or transferred to another system. This is particularly important if you are leasing the system from an application service provider who will be storing your data off-site.

Basis for Cost

Make sure you understand the denominator for cost (e.g., per user, per workstation, per visit, per concurrent user). There may not be a best approach in general, but there probably is a best approach for your situation. For example, if you have many potential users, but few actually using the system at any given time, paying by concurrent users may be more cost effective than paying for each registered user. The vendor, of course, will play the opposite game.

Understand the breadth of your implementation. Who will need access to the system? Will it be just your employees, or will others (such as referring physicians, other healthcare organizations, and patients) need access? Will your vendor allow you to resell use of the software to others?

Maintenance Costs

Try to tie ongoing maintenance costs to some external benchmarks, such as the consumer price index (CPI). While most vendors will not agree to use a straight CPI formula, many will accept CPI plus specified percentage points.

Agree on a written issue-escalation policy with definite time frames for resolution of issues, especially software bug fixes. This is useful over the life of the relationship, but critical during the implementation.

As important as a good contract is, the fact remains that a true partnership is based upon common values and shared success. Before signing a contract, get to know your vendor by way of face-to-face meetings, structured phone interviews, interviews with other customers, and if possible, interviews with organizations that selected a different vendor. In addition, use published vendor ratings (based on questionnaires and interviews with IT leaders of CDOs). KLAS Enterprises, LLC has an extensive listing of customer ratings of healthcare system vendors, including software quality, implementation support and ongoing support (2).

Summary

Our approach to EHR vendor selection focused on assessing how the software could support our strategic goals and operational needs. We focused on large-scale work processes (e.g., scheduling an outpatient appointment, conducting and documenting a clinic visit), rather than reviewing lists of software functions. In this way, the process was very different from the one we use for selecting other information systems (such as those in lab and radiology), for which we develop and score detailed RFPs. We chose a partner that shared our vision for how automation could improve care delivery processes and that could demonstrate the success of its product in environments similar to ours.

References

1. Marsh P. *Contract Negotiations Handbook*. 2nd ed. Gower Publishing Company; 1984.
2. KLAS Enterprises. http://www.healtmputing.com/site/v2/

4
Infrastructure

FRANK RICHARDS

Introduction

A solid foundation is a basic requirement for any structure that is meant to last. Any information system (but particularly an EHR) requires a solid infrastructure that can support the software and its users. This chapter discusses several aspects of information infrastructure, including strategies for avoiding downtimes. Although this is one of the more technical chapters, some members of your team will need to understand these issues—either to manage an outsourcing contract or to run the system internally. Even non-technical readers should find that some sections of the chapter help them understand at a conceptual level how the IT infrastructure supports an effective EHR. The references are provided as examples of the kinds of resources that are available. There may be others that are more suited to your specific questions or needs.

What Is in The Infrastructure?

The infrastructure includes the supporting hardware, software and management systems required to run a particular application or suite of applications (in this case the EHR). This includes the data network (routers, wires, switches, hubs), workstations (PCs, laptops, hand-held devices), servers (database, application, print/file), and telecommunications equipment and services. In most cases, it also includes the controlled environment in which many of these components operate. (Although computer equipment no longer has the rigid requirements for temperature and humidity that it once had, housing your core system components, servers, and communications equipment in controlled, secured areas is still essential for a reliable infrastructure.)

The design and complexity of the infrastructure will depend on the size and complexity of your organization, as well as your ability to function without the EHR should it be unavailable. For mid-sized to large organizations (i.e., those with hundreds or thousands of users) falling back on manual processes when the automated system is down is problematic at best, and, in the worst case, may compromise patient care.

The Network

All systems that support more than a single user require a local area network (LAN) to allow different users to access the features, functions and data in the EHR. LANs come in different configurations and can use different communication protocols. Currently, most organizations use transmission control protocol/internet protocol (TCP/IP) over Ethernet for their LAN environment. TCP/IP was originally developed for the Department of Defense and is the basis for communicating on the Internet. Discussing the nature of these protocols in any technical detail is beyond the scope of this book. A basic technical overview of TCP/IP and other network protocols can be found at http://www.yale.edu/pclt/COMM/TCPIP.HTM.

Networks vary greatly in their complexity, depending on size and scope. The number of nodes, the amount of data being transferred and the number of users all contribute to network load, and to the demand for network capacity (bandwidth). It is important that your network be sized properly (i.e., deliver adequate bandwidth) for your applications to operate at acceptable speeds. If you are running multiple applications from different vendors, you will need more bandwidth. Most large and mid-size organizations have a network in place before implementing an EHR. However, the existing network infrastructure may have insufficient capacity and reliability to support an EHR, particularly if the EHR incorporates very large files, such as radiology images, scanned documents and voice files. These require substantially more bandwidth than typical support systems (such as laboratory and pharmacy) do.

If your organization includes multiple sites separated by more than a few thousand feet, or in cases where you cannot obtain the right-of-way necessary to install your own communication (e.g., cable or fiber optics), you will need to consider a wide-area network (WAN) architecture. WAN services vary by geographic location and are usually purchased from a telecommunications company, such as AT&T, Pacific Bell or Verizon. Capacity (bandwidth) for a WAN is generally much more expensive than comparable LAN capacity, so cost can become the primary constraint to extending applications to widely separated practices. This problem is more acute in a rural setting, but can be a consideration in urban settings as well. There are many WAN services available, with more options becoming available, but the cost of WAN connectivity is still at least an order of magnitude greater than for a LAN. This makes network design more challenging and more complicated. For example, traffic prioritization and scheduling of large file transfers and downloads are not typically necessary in a LAN environment where bandwidth is plentiful. In a WAN environment, traffic-generating activities need to be assessed up front and prioritized or scheduled appropriately to insure that critical applications will have sufficient bandwidth to provide users with acceptable response times.

At Geisinger, we deal with about 50 physical locations located in 31 rural counties, many of which lack the telecommunications options found in urban areas. We run applications on servers in the corporate data center and deliver them to other parts of the system using services leased from several telephone and cable companies. Because of the wide variety of applications and services that we offer, and the relatively high cost of WAN bandwidth, we employ several delivery methods:

Wide-Area Bandwidth

We deliver connectivity to most sites using T1 or T3 lines leased from one or more local telephone companies. A typical connection speed is 1.5 megabits per second, which provides adequate capacity for the EHR, E-mail, and other necessary systems, such as the lab information system, and browser-based applications. This connection speed is not sufficient for applications that require large bandwidth (such as print and file sharing that map a server's hard drive) or that transfer very large files, such as some PC maintenance operations. Traditional Picture Archiving and Communication

Systems (PACS) used to store and move radiology images can easily overwhelm a T1, as can multiple Internet surfers.

Newer network equipment with more sophisticated traffic prioritization algorithms is helping to address these issues. Routers and bandwidth-shaping tools can be used to prioritize traffic by type (e.g., HTTP, Telnet), source, destination (IP address), or simply by the amount of bandwidth being used. The latter technique is the one we use most. Traffic that begins to occupy large amounts of bandwidth is automatically throttled back and prevented from consuming the entire network. We use a number of criteria to prioritize traffic, but the first principle is that access to the EHR takes priority over other functions.

Local Servers

Local servers are used where there is a need to support server-based file and print sharing, especially for local printers. Inexpensive servers provide print and file sharing at each location and local disk space for large files that need to be accessed regularly.

Remote Client Hosting

Another technique to limit bandwidth requirements is to run the client software (programs that normally run locally on the user's PC) on one or more servers centrally located in a secure facility. The user's PC only needs to perform the screen formatting and keyboard, mouse, and cursor movements. For many applications that require a "fat" client (one that has a large number of programs), this can significantly decrease network bandwidth requirements and allow remote users to run an application over a WAN that would normally require the high speeds of a LAN. However, depending on the applications and communication protocol used, this remote hosting can actually increase network bandwidth requirements. For example, moving a text-based application to a remote hosting arrangement using Telnet as the communications protocol could increase bandwidth requirements. Whether remote hosting is cost-effective in your environment will depend on the nature of the applications, the bandwidth each requires, the number of concurrent users per remote server, how often you upgrade your computer hardware and software, and the cost of WAN bandwidth.

Geisinger uses remote hosting for its EHR application suite to manage software upgrades efficiently, to increase the useful life of PC's and—in some cases—to minimize bandwidth requirements at remote sites. This approach allows us to use a five-year life cycle for PCs. It also makes it feasible to use telephone lines for emergency back-up connectivity for some remote practices.

Other Ways to Connect

In addition to leased services from telephone companies, we use other methods of connecting to remote practices, including cable modems, ISDN, and wireless (radio). Most of these alternates are deployed as a back-up to the primary leased service. They operate at much slower speeds (usually in the 128 to 750 kilobits/second range). We estimate that using our EHR requires 60 kilobits/second/device of bandwidth for brisk response times.

In cities, high-speed bandwidth may be available in the form of a metropolitan area network (MAN). MAN bandwidth is generally less costly per megabyte than the comparable WAN capacity, but is usually only cost-effective where there is a high population density in a small geographical area. We have been able to create a MAN that extends approximately eight miles from the main campus. This allows us to connect several of our local administrative offices to a high-speed backbone, providing campus-like LAN network speed. (Normally, these offices would require WAN connections, since they are too far away to connect to the campus LAN). We use "dark fiber" from the local cable TV company for the MAN. It allows us to use our own networking hardware and can achieve bandwidths of up to 4 gigabits per second. An added advantage to this approach is that you can start with relatively inexpensive equipment and scale up as more bandwidth is needed—although convincing a local carrier to rent you space on their network may be difficult.

Redundancy

Because we host our applications centrally, reliable network connectivity is crucial to system availability. On our two large campuses we use parallel networks to provide near 100% availability. Half of the PCs in each hospital unit and hospital-based practice are connected to each network (see Figure 4.1). This means that the loss of one network will leave functioning PCs in every clinical area. Another approach is to have dual network paths to every PC (i.e., workstations with two network cards). This allows all PCs to continue to operate if either network is lost. It also doubles the cost of the network, limiting its use to critical settings that have limited space for redundant PCs.

Today's networks are more than just miles of cable connecting terminal devices to host computers. They are highly complex computer systems in their own right, and as such require special expertise to design, implement and maintain. Many organizations find it more cost-effective to outsource this area of IT. Whether or not that makes sense for you will depend on your size, location, and availability of network experts. We have chosen thus far to keep most of our technical support—including the network staff—in house, partly because of our size and geographic location, and partly because benchmarking shows it to be more cost-effective.

Wireless LANs

While wireless networks may not replace their wired cousins in the near term, they offer an effective way for mobile workers to stay connected to their applications. One can easily envision a busy clinician carrying a pen tablet computer from her home to a rehab facility and then to a community hospital external to Geisinger, having access to the latest clinical information on patients all along the way. Although this is an attractive vision, there are a few issues with wireless LAN's that you should consider before you implement this structure. They are security, bandwidth, battery life, cost, size and the durability of mobile devices.

A wireless network is, by its nature, less secure then its tethered counterpart because some level of authentication is implicit in gaining physical access to a computer connected to the network. The biggest risk early adopters of wireless LAN's encountered was the lack of security. Like the signals from early cordless phones and analog cell phones, signals from wireless networks were easily intercepted. There are many disturbing stories in the industry about networks that were entered by people sitting in the company parking lot. While security for wireless networks has improved, in 2004 there is still no one, easily applied, robust security standard. Several competing security schemes are being developed, but it is not clear which will become dominant.

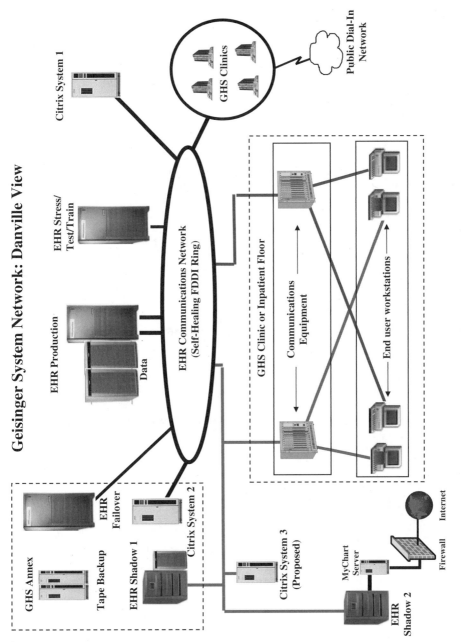

Geisinger System Network: Danville View

FIGURE 4.1. Network architecture to guarantee her access.

Despite these drawbacks, it is likely that wireless will play an increasingly important role in healthcare IT systems. The mobility afforded by wireless is too compelling for it to be ignored.

At the very least, ensure that a user is authenticated before receiving a wireless connection and that data is encrypted more securely than the Wired-Equivalent Privacy (WEP) feature of commodity wireless devices can accomplish. WEP is vulnerable because of the relatively short initialization vector (IV) used in its encryption process. It has a number of shortcomings and its encryption keys can easily be discovered by tools such as NetStumbler® and Airsnort®. These "sniffers" monitor and analyze network traffic and recover encryption keys. This makes WEP especially vulnerable in large networks that generate large volumes of traffic.

Despite these shortcomings, WEP is the necessary foundation for wireless security. Stronger security measures are available using port-based authentication and key distribution. These require additional hardware and software, and are more complex to configure and deploy. But given the ease of breaking the WEP encryption scheme, additional security measures are usually required to avoid network break-ins and protect patient information. For more information about wireless network security, see http://www.wi-fiplanet.com/tutorials/article.php/2233511.

Personal Computers

From the outset, IT professionals were unimpressed with PCs. They seemed like toys, with inferior computing power, limited functionality, inferior operating systems, and virtually no security. Twenty years later, the operating system interface and functionality have improved, but PCs remain hard to manage and protect. Though there are many PC management tools available, they still lag behind similar utilities found on mainframe and server-based systems. These security and software management challenges are particularly worrisome in the case of an EHR because of the sensitive nature of the data and the need of users for highly reliable access. Here are some suggestions to manage your desktop environment:

Deploy a Standard Desktop

This is particularly useful in areas where individual PCs are shared by multiple users (e.g., exam rooms, clinic front desk areas). Standards for software, desktop layout (including colors and screen backgrounds) and directory structures will help users move easily from one machine to another, decreasing calls to the Help Desk. Until recently, locking down PC system configurations was a time-consuming task, especially if more than a few hundred devices were involved. Newer products from Microsoft and others are making the task easier. We dedicate about 10 FTE staff to maintain the configuration of approximately 8,000 PCs.

Deploy Remote PC-Management Software

Dispatching people to fix problems on-site is costly and time-consuming in all but the smallest settings. Most mid-sized and large-sized CDOs occupy at least a large building or a campus. At Geisinger, the IT desktop support staff covers over fifty sites in 31 counties. And, although we station support staff regionally, sending a technician to a practice to fix a simple PC problem is expensive. With the user's permission, we use software that allows the technician to take control of the user device remotely. This allows the technician to do and see everything as if they were sitting in front of the PC, dramatically reducing the time needed to troubleshoot desktop problems and allowing us to support our PCs with 20 FTE technicians. It also means that the user is able to resume work far more quickly. Even if you outsource this function, you should ask your outsourcer if they have this capability. It will ultimately save your users' time and your organization money.

In addition to decreasing break/fix cycle time, many PC-management packages contain modules that maintain software inventories, allowing remote updating of desktop software. This saves time and resources when new versions of software need to be loaded on PCs. However, potential problems with these programs need attention. First, many of these systems work best with a standard directory structure. If your users have moved or changed files or renamed directories, it will be difficult to automate the software process without causing additional, manual effort. Second, preparing a software "package" is complicated by the need to deal with PCs that contain software not tested or supported by the organization. There are also nuances to the software installation process that only become apparent with automated updating of hundreds or thousands of machines. For example, a software update might fail because a particular file is not where the program or script expects it to be. When a human operator loads software from a CD, they can respond effectively to most error situations. Automated software updates require that the update's author anticipate as many error situations as possible and design appropriate responses. At the least, the error must be documented for further follow up. At best you would like the update program to resolve the error automatically. But under no circumstances do you want the update program to do anything harmful to the PC. The best approach is to test repeatedly before deployment.

Testing Desktop Software

Most organizations have a mixed PC environment. Different platforms (i.e., versions of operating systems), machine types and speeds, and different combinations of applications make desktop management a challenge. For example, PC-management software may not work well—or at all—on some platforms. To further complicate matters, there is usually a variety of programs running in the background (virus checkers, printer drivers and other utility programs).

One important way to reduce the risk associated with rolling out new versions of software is to create a real-world test environment. The size and complexity of your computing environment will determine the size and complexity of your test bench. In general, it should include most of the hardware and software configurations found in your organization. Its main purpose is to uncover conflicts and incompatibilities that may arise among your various system components.

Home PCs

More and more clinicians require access to clinical information from home using their own PCs. Different organizations approach support of these PCs in different ways, but support always poses a special set of challenges. You will have no control over who uses these PCs, what software is installed, how they connect to the Internet or how vulnerable they are to attacks. We provide strictly limited support for these PCs.

We do not (for example) send technicians to employees' homes to assist with problems. At the same time, we have designed our infrastructure to minimize support needs. Below are some of ways we have attempted to manage this complex environment.

Access: There are a number of ways to provide remote access to the CDO's network. These include direct dial-in to a modem pool hosted by the CDO, dial-in to an Internet Service Provider (ISP), broadband Internet access via digital subscriber line (DSL) from the phone company, and broadband access via cable modem. The connection established with direct dial-in to the CDO is inherently more secure than any of the other alternatives because it does not pass over the Internet, and is, therefore, harder to intercept. The disadvantage is that the organization bears the cost of the dial-in hardware and staff to maintain the system and user accounts.

Having users connect to the modem pool through an ISP (using dial-up, DSL or cable modem) has the advantage of getting the healthcare organization out of the modem-pool business, but requires additional security measures.

Security: To establish a secure connection you will need to implement one or more additional layers of software to provide encryption and authentication. Our encryption methods include IPsec (IP security protocol—a protocol for negotiating encryption and authentication at the IP host level), virtual private networks (VPNs), secure-socket-layer (SSL) 128-bit encryption, and tokens (key-fob sized devices that provide access codes that are synchronized with the security server). Other available methods are public key encryption (PKI) using digital certificates residing on the PC, smartcards and other physical devices. These methods tend to be more complex to set up and administer than tokens. Though an in-depth discussion of security techniques is beyond the scope of this chapter, here are a few things to consider when deciding on a security scheme for home access users.

VPN software is a very secure method of connecting users over the Internet, but it requires users to have either special hardware or software loaded on their remote PC. Whenever users load new software on their home PC, you run the risk of creating software incompatibilities, since you cannot know the environment into which the new software is being introduced. We reserve VPN for users skilled enough to deal with issues that may arise or when there is no other reasonable alternative. Done correctly (especially over a broadband connection), a VPN allows the user to work from home with system response times that closely mimic the LAN.

Currently, our preferred method of providing secure home access uses SSL and a hardware token that generates a new access code in sync with the server every 60 seconds. The user must have a password and a token-generated code to connect to the network. All that is required on the user's home PC is a browser capable of supporting SSL with 128-bit encryption (see Figure 4.2). In this scenario, applications that are not browser-based are published via a server (in our case using Citrix® from Citrix Systems, Inc). This allows the application to run remotely at the host site, only downloading a small client application (Java applet) to the PC, minimizing the risk of software conflicts.

Supporting desktop PCs continues to be a management challenge for IT departments. The original paradigm of the "personal computer," with special purpose software and locally stored data, is alive and well in most organizations. This is particularly true of CDOs, which need many different software applications to support their many work processes, which routinely span patient care, administration, research and teaching. Providing all of these applications in a server-based environment is usually not

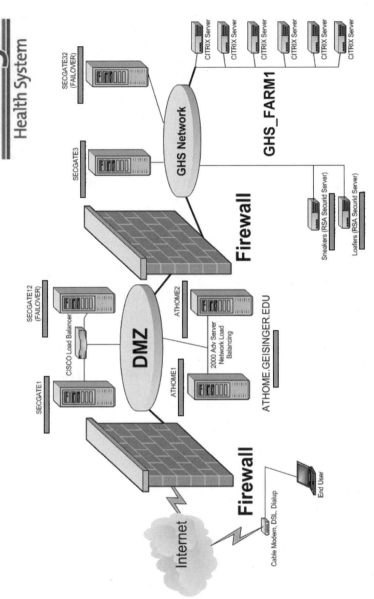

FIGURE 4.2. Geisinger at home.

practical, since each application requires time to set up, test and maintain. In the near-term, employing desktop management systems and enforcing unifying standards is probably the best way to manage this environment.

Backup and Recover: How Much Security Is Enough?

It has been said that the only thing on earth that works every time is gravity. No matter how carefully a system is designed, tested and implemented, there will be times when the system is unavailable, either by plan or by accident. Planning for downtime is an important part of the overall implementation of any IT system but is particularly important when implementing an EHR. The better your organization gets at using the EHR to improve patient care, the harder working without it becomes. We've talked about some ways to provide a stable, well-managed environment. You will also want to develop and test policies, procedures and technologies that will let you continue to function when the EHR is unavailable. We have developed a number of processes to deal with downtimes, both planned and unplanned.

Have a Plan to Give EHR Users the Information They Need

There are a number of potential scenarios in which the EHR will be unavailable. The specific design of your system will determine your most frequent causes of downtime—loss of the main server, a major network outage, or power loss to an entire site. The method for mitigating the impact of each problem differs, but the goal is always to keep user operations as normal as possible. The amount of time, effort and money you decide to invest should be proportional to your level of risk, and the time, effort and money you lose when the system is unavailable. Anderson (1), in a careful study, calculated that an hour of downtime costs a 500-bed hospital $15,800 in added labor costs alone. This means that an EHR system that is available 97% of the time (that is, unavailable 263 hours a year) would cost $2.8 million a year more in salaries than a system with a 99% uptime (which would be unavailable 88 hours a year). It also means that even 99% uptime represents a labor cost of $1.4 million a year (See Figure 4.3).

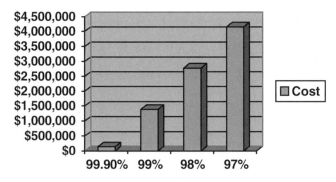

FIGURE 4.3. Annual labor costs of EHR downtime in a 500-bed hospital.

Preventing Host Server Outages

Downtimes related to failure of a central (host) server can be most disruptive, especially if the downtime is due to a hardware failure that produces database errors. Having a tested back-up and restore plan is essential. Below are the specific steps we have taken to address the issue of a central server failure.

- A back-up server that is running a shadow (or back-up) copy of the EHR (a so-called "hot spare") is available at all times should the main server fail. This server is used for training and testing purposes when not needed to run the production EHR. We practice failing over to this server periodically to insure that the staff know the procedure and can complete their tasks in the shortest time possible.
- All data is stored redundantly on two separate storage disk subsystems (Redundant Array of Inexpensive Disks—RAID 5). The systems are located in separate secure areas.
- A shadow copy of the EHR is continually updated with the latest transactions from the production EHR server. The shadow system consists of a server and disk array, and provides an up-to-the-minute, alternate source of all EHR data. The shadow system cannot be updated directly by the users, and is used for data retrieval only. It is, however, always available and can be immediately accessed if the main system fails. It is also used as a means to off-load some database searching and reporting activity from the main server, increasing the main server's capacity and improving EHR response times.
- Tape back-ups are performed nightly, so that in the event of a disaster the information on tape is never more than 24 hours old.
- At sites connected to the main server via the WAN, summary EHR information on patients who are scheduled to be seen the next day is downloaded to a PC located in the practice every night. This information allows the practice to function with minimal disruption in the event of central server or network downtimes.

Primary Network Outages

Outages due to network connectivity loss fall into two categories, wide-area and local-area (WAN and LAN, respectively). We have discussed these earlier in this chapter and have also discussed some of the issues related to each. In general, LANs can be made more reliable because they don't rely on a third party (e.g., a phone company) to operate.

Current statistics from our EHR system show about 0.01% unscheduled downtime due to main system failure, and 0.76% total downtime (both scheduled and unscheduled). Partial outages due to network failures are more difficult to characterize, as they usually affect only a limited number of users (e.g., a particular practice, or building). Overall network connectivity problems result in about 3.3% unscheduled downtime and occur most frequently at WAN-connected sites.

Some steps we have taken to provide high availability connectivity to our sites include:

- On our two acute-care campuses we use parallel networks to achieve high availability (Figure 4.4). While parallel networks are critical for acute-care sites, they are too expensive to be deployed in most outpatient practices, where the environment is simpler and more stable.
- We have implemented a highly segmented, switched network design, which provides dedicated bandwidth, along with a routed core to prevent large segments of the

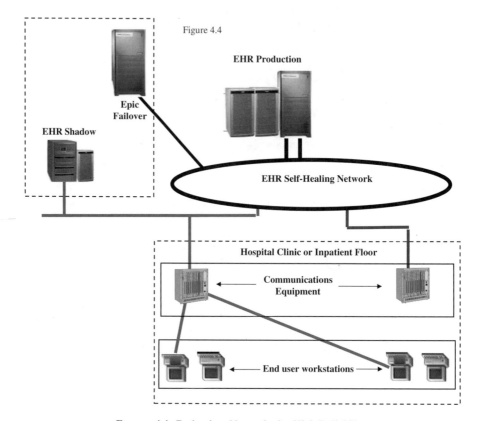

FIGURE 4.4. Redundant Networks for High Reliability.

network from being affected by adverse network events (e.g., "broadcast storms" and other events that produce high levels of network traffic). This design allows problems to be isolated quickly and prevents unwanted traffic from affecting major portions of the network. A recent, highly publicized, multi-day system outage at a major U.S. teaching hospital was the result of a network architecture that was not optimal for its high volume environment. The network was heavily dependent on bridging (as opposed to routing), making it more vulnerable in times of excessively high traffic. When a network problem created high traffic volumes (a "broadcast storm"), the traffic volume made accessing applications impossible and diagnosing the root problem difficult.

Your network design needs to be suited to your environment, and environments change over time. Plan to monitor your traffic volumes and re-assess your network needs at least annually.

- Our wide-area services are generally based on leased lines (i.e., T-1, T-3). We use ISDN, cable modem or DSL services to back up the leased lines. Unfortunately, except in the case of cable modems, these services are delivered by the same provider using the same physical routes as the leased lines. Adverse events that affect the main connection can also affect the back-up line.

- Finally, in order to cope with a major disaster, such as losing the main Data Center, we have created two separate connections to the telephone network, each in a separate building at opposite ends of the campus. This minimizes the risk that we will be cut off from the telephone carrier's network in the event of a disaster. For useful sources of additional information, see: NetworkWorld or www.nwfusion.com).

Preventing Power Loss

As with network connectivity, outages due to power loss are easier to prevent on the major campuses, where generator power and battery back-up are widely available. Some steps to take to avoid power loss:

- Provide UPS (Uninterruptible Power Source) protection and generator back-up to all data centers (manned or unmanned).
- Provide UPS protection for all communication closets so they can withstand short outages of up to 15–30 minutes without losing connectivity. This includes all practice sites, as well as inpatient facilities. (UPSs that will provide longer protection are available and may be appropriate in specific settings, but are expensive).
- A laptop computer with a fresh battery can enable a practice to function despite power loss. Many of our remote practices use one or two laptops for on-call physicians, as well as this back-up function.

How much resource you allocate to back-up and recovery depends upon the costs your organization incurs when the EHR is unavailable. At a minimum, you should have a backup strategy that allows you to recover your data in a timely manner and does not put you at risk for losing all your patients' records. It is wise to keep a daily backup of your system in a location other than where the system itself resides. Then, if your hardware system is destroyed, you can recreate it on new hardware. Also remember that total recovery time includes any time it takes to get replacement hardware and software, as well as the time required to enter any data that was generated after the last back-up was made. (See: www.internetnews.com for more details.)

Data Security: Can You Protect Your Data from the World's Bad People?

Cyber attacks have been escalating at an alarming rate. Viruses, worms, denial of service attacks and identity theft have made headlines in trade magazines, as well as the mainstream press. If your organization is connected to the Internet, you are vulnerable. The good news is that there are many ways to protect your organization's data. The bad news is they require time, money, and constant monitoring.

Firewalls

Every CDO that connects to the Internet should do so through a firewall. Firewalls work by filtering the information flowing into and out of an organization. They protect the PCs on the company's network by acting as a gateway, which hides the identity of the individual workstations, thus making them difficult to discover from the Internet. Firewalls use one or more methods to filter unwanted traffic.

- Packet filtering: Packets (small chunks of data) are analyzed and compared to a set of filters. Filters may include TCP/IP addresses, domain name and communication protocols. Packets that make it through the filters are sent to the receiving system. All others are discarded.

- Proxy service: A proxy service acts as a mediator between the workstation and the Internet. Information from the Internet is retrieved by the firewall and then sent to the requesting PC and vice versa. This hides the identity of the PC from the Internet, reducing the risk of attacks directly to the PC. This makes defending against attacks somewhat easier, since the PC identity (or IP address) is not accessible.
- Stateful inspection: This is a newer method in which the certain key components of each packet are compared to a database of trusted information. Information traveling from inside the firewall to the Internet is monitored for specific defining characteristics. Incoming information is then compared to these characteristics. If the comparison yields a reasonable match, the information is allowed through. Otherwise it is discarded.

Large organizations deploy multiple firewalls to handle the volume of traffic and the complex filters required for various types of business. Multiple firewalls are also useful in establishing one or more demilitarized zones (see Figure 4.2). A DMZ further separates your internal network from external networks, and prevents Internet sources from directly referencing your internal systems. The DMZ creates a buffer area that protects servers that you want people on the Internet to be able to reach, while keeping those servers separate from your internal, mission-critical systems. (Further information is available at www.sans.org.)

Antivirus Protection

A virus is a computer program designed to make copies, or replicate itself. It is this replication that makes it a virus. It may or may not do damage to your computer. Viruses are spread (intentionally or unintentionally) by people (e.g., through E-mail). Unlike viruses, worms are designed to spread from computer to computer without the aid of humans. This is why worms spread much more quickly than viruses. The third form of "malware" is the Trojan horse, which appears to have one purpose, but really does something else. For purposes of this discussion, we will use the term virus to refer to all forms of malware. Further information about viruses, trojans and worms is freely available. (2)

There are numerous systems and software products that offer virus protection. We use a three-tiered virus protection strategy to catch suspect programs as early as possible. An initial scan of all incoming E-mail is performed to look for suspicious attachments. Recently we have begun stripping off all executable attachments (an attachment containing a small computer program that includes instructions for the computer to follow) from incoming E-mail in an effort to further minimize exposure to malicious programs. Next, internal servers search for viruses and worms. Finally, each individual PC scans incoming files and E-mail attachments, as well as running a complete scan of itself weekly. This approach has led to quick isolation of suspicious programs and minimized damage to our systems. In some cases, it still is not fast enough to prevent "infections." When infected PCs or servers are identified, they are isolated from the network and "cleaned" using appropriate software.

Intrusion Detection and External Testing

Intrusion detection and external testing are additional proactive security measures aimed at spotting the bad guys before they can do damage. A network intrusion detection system (NIDS) looks at packets of data as they cross the network, looking for tell-tale signs of hacking. These systems may also monitor system files and log files looking for signs that these files have been modified. Until recently, intrusion detection systems have been of limited value, as hackers were generally more advanced than the systems trying to detect them. Newer systems using more sophisticated methods of intrusion detection are now available. They offer higher levels of protection.

The price of protection is variable, from a few hundred dollars to tens of thousands (or even millions of dollars for very large companies). The right combination of products and systems will depend on the complexity and size of your organization, as well as the risk hackers pose to your business, but being connected to the Internet with no protection is an invitation to hackers that you can be sure they will accept.

Summary

As the foundation of the EHR, IT infrastructure has been raised to a new level of importance and organizational visibility. Reliable connectivity, well-managed desktops, solid back-up procedures, and protection from those who might intentionally or unintentionally do harm to your organization's information systems must be primary areas of focus if you intend to deliver timely information around-the-clock.

If you are responsible for developing and maintaining the technical environment, be sure that you have allowed for adequate resources, training, and any outside help you may need. If you are outsourcing, be sure your vendor has all of the necessary personnel, systems and safeguards in place to keep you up and running. No matter how well designed and managed your systems and their underpinnings may be, there will be times when they fail. Clear downtime plans, policies, and procedures will enable you to continue to operate with a minimum of disruption to your business.

References

1. Anderson M. The Toll Of Downtime: A Study Calculates the Time and Money Lost When Automated Systems Go Down. Healthcare Informatics April 2002.
2. Symantec Inc. www.symantec.com/avcenter/reference/worm.vs.virus.pdf.

Additional Reading

For more detailed information, trade journals and the Internet are excellent sources of information. All major computer publications (e.g., COMPUTERWORLD, InformationWeek, NetworkWorld and InfoWorld) are good sources to track industry trends on the topics discussed here. Most have electronic versions or e-mail synopses of current issues. Internet search engines such as Google (http://www.google.com) are powerful tools that can help you locate information on general and specific topics. The URLs presented in this chapter are only examples of the wealth of information that is available on the Internet. Just watch out for viruses!

5
Workflow Assessment and Redesign

Jean A. Adams, Linda M. Culp, and Janet S. Byron

Introduction

To implement an EHR effectively, operational leaders and implementation teams will need to understand your organization's current workflows. This understanding will guide your needs assessments for the implementation and provide the starting point for redesigning more efficient work processes. We concentrate on designing EHR workflows that facilitate clinical best practice, rather than automating existing workflows, believing that this approach produces greater improvements in efficiency and quality. Other care-delivery organizations (CDOs) focus on automating existing flow to simplify the implementation. We are not aware of any but anecdotal evidence regarding which approach is preferable. Most organizations probably take a blended approach, based on multiple local factors.

After our high-level vision teams and process redesign teams developed needs assessments and optimal clinical practices that could be supported by the EHR (see Chapter 2), subgroups of the process redesign teams analyzed existing practice workflows and recommended specific workflows that would optimize safety, quality, efficiency, and patient satisfaction. The full redesign team evaluated these recommendations and adjusted workflows, as appropriate. The EHR oversight team approved these new workflows.

The following workflows were similar across varying practices:

- Charts pulls and refiling of charts
- Service sheet completion
- Paper medical record preparation
- Preparation of test results for physician signature
- Filing of test results in the paper medical record
  - Billing charge entry
  - Documentation of office visits and resulting on-site testing

The next step was to customize the new workflows to accommodate the unique needs of each individual practice. For example, some practices use Geisinger laboratory services almost exclusively, while others use outside labs. These differences necessitated variations in the order management and test result filing workflows.

To prepare for each practice's implementation, the team filled out the Site Characteristics Questionnaire (Appendix 5). A data analyst then completed a workflow analysis customized for small, medium and large practices (See Figure 5.1).

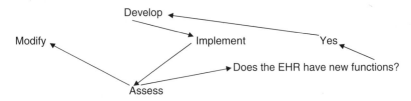

FIGURE 5.1. The redesign process was iterative, moving successively through four phases: (1) development, (2) implementation, (3) assessment, and (4) modification.

One month after go-live, we conducted post-implementation assessments through questionnaires and direct observation of the implemented workflows in practice. This feedback led to further workflow modifications. Subsequent feedback and modification loops are completed by way of informal communication (typically E-mails) among practice managers, clinicians, and the implementation team.

An example of the assessment of the impact of one workflow re-design is illustrated in Figure 5.2. Ten steps were eliminated, while 5 others were improved.

As the EHR software is upgraded, workflows must be reviewed. This review helps identify whether new software functions should be used and, secondarily, which workflows can be further improved. We regularly decide not to use new EHR software functions because they do not support our preferred workflows. (The ability to choose not to implement new software functions is little discussed but is an important determinant of the EHR's value.) Workflow review and redesign may also be prompted by the implementation of additional software products (other applications of the EHR suite or special purpose software) and by the implementation of new interfaces to other information systems.

Unexpectedly, our redesigned workflows were applicable to most practices without significant variation. Analysis revealed only minor differences between primary care and specialty practices. The similarities of many workflows, allowed us to move to a system of piloting new workflows in a single practice preparatory to a rapid system-wide roll out. These pilots provide adequate testing of the workflows and further modifications are not usually needed.

After three years, we disbanded the centralized process redesign teams and shifted the responsibility for process improvement to individual implementation teams. This was partly due to the fact that using the EHR implementation as an opportunity for workflow improvement had become widely accepted. It was also an acknowledgement of the fact that workflow improvement is most effective when it is led by clinical and operational leaders.

Oversight

Two forums validate new EHR workflows that either need multidisciplinary review or that have the potential for CDO-wide effects. The first is a multidisciplinary feedback team comprised of physicians, nurses, ancillary staff, IT personnel, and professional reimbursement staff. The second team is comprised of operations leaders (including financial personnel) from throughout the organization. These teams review proposed workflows and communicate changes to their constituents. The feedback team meets weekly during the height of the implementation, decreasing to monthly

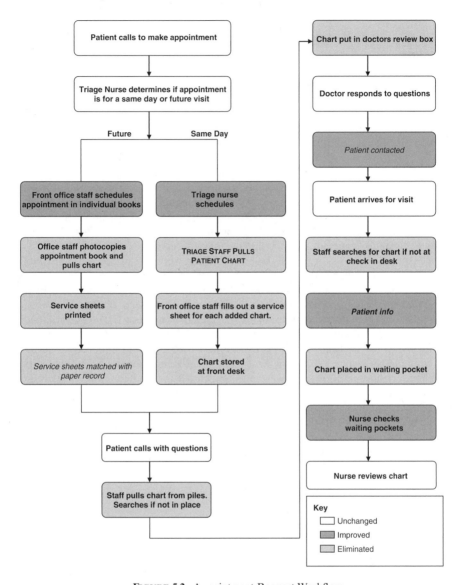

FIGURE 5.2. Appointment Request Workflow.

postimplementation. They review many workflow proposals at most meetings. The operations staff group reviews a major proposal about quarterly.

At times, we form special purpose committees to address specific workflow design needs. For example, we formed a healthcare-team integration committee to define required workflows for physician supervision of midlevel providers, nurses, technicians, residents and students (see Chapter 10).

Summary

1. Consider workflow redesign as a potential benefit of EHR implementation.
2. Involve all the stakeholders early and often.
3. Pilot workflows: Begin at one or two initial sites with careful assessment and modification of workflows.
4. Do not underestimate the resources required.
5. Remember that paper can contribute to an optimal workflow, particularly if it does not need to be filed.

6
Staffing and Managing Implementation Teams

JEAN A. ADAMS and LINDA M. CULP

This chapter outlines methods for staffing your implementation roll-out, including defining the skill sets you will need, identifying people who have or can develop these skills, and managing the multiple teams that will be needed for a large implementation.

As the needs of our implementation project and our understanding of the implementation process have changed, so has our approach to staffing. Our structure has evolved from a few teams staffed by IT generalists to many teams staffed by specialists who serve a specific role (e.g., workflow analyst, trainer) on multiple teams. The team structure that you develop—based on the scope of your implementation, your organization's culture, and the availability of skilled people—will be unique. This chapter is intended to help you plan (and evolve) more effectively.

Physician Champion

We found it very useful to identify a physician champion. The skill set of our first physician champion included:

- The respect of other physicians in the organization
- A vision for automating healthcare
- The ability to communicate the vision to all stakeholders (executives, board members, physicians, IT staff)
- The ability to organize and lead a multidisciplinary feedback team
- An understanding of current workflows and workflow redesign
- The ability to identify and assist physicians struggling to adjust to the EHR

This physician champion, an experienced clinical leader, was named "Vice President (VP), Medical Informatics" and was paired with the CIO. Together, they were responsible for the overall EHR implementation. The CIO oversaw the technical aspects of the implementation (e.g., system stability and scalability). The physician champion was responsible for clinical aspects, such as optimization of clinical workflows and care quality improvement.

Although a physician champion is appropriately cited as being an important factor for a successful implementation (1), relatively little attention is paid to the skills which make a physician champion effective. As an EHR project matures (or extends beyond one hospital) what is probably needed is not so much a single leader as a coordinated group of physician champions. Perhaps one part of the explanation of the high rate of failure of EHR projects is that too frequently the physician champion is required to champion the project alone.

As our implementation has matured, we have refined our understanding of physician champions. The Chief Medical Information Officer (CMIO) and others have identified, educated and empowered physicians throughout the organization to champion the EHR in multiple ways:

- Work closely with the implementation team to implement the practice.
- Design useful EHR tools. (This work is shared by physician informaticians, the CMIO, clinical domain experts, clinical domain experts (see Chapter 9), physician members of multidisciplinary feedback groups, and the virtual feedback group (or VFG; see Chapter 18).
- Provide informed feedback on EHR effectiveness (physician informaticians, domain experts, CORUM, VFG, and the CMIO).
- Provide executive physician leadership (CMIO, CEO, Chief Medical Officer (CMO), Associate CMOs).
- Create and communicate a vision for using information systems to improve healthcare (CMIO, CEO, CMO, physician informaticians, CORUM).
- Lead departments in ongoing process redesign and EHR optimization (domain experts, Associate CMOs, CMIO, physician informaticians).
- Identify, educate and coordinate physician champions (CMIO, Clinical leaders, physician informaticians).

Even in smaller practices of 10 physicians or less, aim for shared physician contributions to your EHR implementation.

The First Teams

The first project team consisted of a Senior Systems Analyst, a Senior Management Engineer, two Senior Technical Analysts, and two System Analysts. As the implementation extended to increasing numbers of practices, the project team expanded from six to 24 people. An IT project director was assigned to oversee the project. The interface, network design, and technical support teams reported to other directors in IT and ultimately to the CIO. The twelve systems analysts on the implementation team also had a dual reporting relationship, to the project director and to the leaders of the individual practices. Over time, we found that practices preferred for the project director to supervise the analysts and manage the implementation in close consultation with the practice's leaders.

To manage the rapid increase in practice implementations, we also engaged consultants to supplement our analysts. Although the consultants were capable, we found that they did not meet our needs. They did not understand our organizational culture, IT standards, EHR system set-up, or how we integrate the EHR with other applications. They were also expensive, and were often unavailable when most needed. After six months, we replaced the consultants with new hires from nursing, laboratory, and our business office, as well as from outside the organization. The internal people had deep knowledge of our organization. All of the new hires received intensive, standardized training (see below). Most have become long-term contributors to the project.

After we completed implementation in our primary care practices, our focus shifted to the specialty practices. At first, a single analyst did the workflow analysis, planned the EHR system build (see Glossary), customized practice workflows, and trained users. While this approach had the virtues of simplicity and continuity, it also had serious weaknesses. The extended timeline it entailed meant that some practices had difficulty maintaining focus on the project. Worse, since all the IT knowledge of the project resided with one person, that person's absence could create a crisis. On one occasion, the analyst became unavailable the night before a practice went live. This required one of our best analysts to drop all other responsibilities in order to learn the details of the implementation and support the go-live.

Implementing specialty practices rapidly created a number of benefits. Primary care physicians were impatient to use the EHR to coordinate patients' care with specialists. The sooner all clinical notes were in the EHR, the sooner we could stop pulling the paper chart for every office visit and patient telephone call. (Until that time, the paper chart had to be reviewed to guarantee that no significant new observation had been recorded in it.) For these reasons, the EHR Project Oversight Committee (comprised of operational and IT leaders) decided that our 70 specialty and subspecialty clinics should be implemented over 18 months.

Since we had too few experienced analysts to support this scale of implementation using the single-analyst model, we then created a new staffing model, with implementation teams led by experienced analysts and largely comprised of temporary staff and members of a flexible staffing pool.

Temporary Staff

The temporary staff are full-time, salaried employees. Given our rural location, and the fact that the positions are temporary, we provide full benefits to attract qualified applicants. The candidate pool includes IT veterans displaced in the dot-com bust, new college graduates looking for an entry-level position, and Geisinger employees who want to work on the EHR project. The selection process includes an interview and an assessment of analytical and computer skills. We look for people who have a positive "can do" attitude, good communication skills, and the ability to think outside the box. Over time, most of these employees have become full-time.

Flexible Staff

Flexible staff employees are paid an hourly rate that is significantly higher than minimum wage. They do not receive benefits and work on an "as needed" basis. They provide supplemental project support (for example, shadow training). They also serve as a source of trained replacements to fill temporary and permanent positions. They are generally college students (including some who are doing internships), recent graduates looking for IT experience, and displaced IT veterans willing to use the position as a stepping stone to a permanent position.

Training

New team members complete a training curriculum that covers the EHR's software configuration, workflow analysis and redesign, and user training and support in 16 hours of classroom training, three weeks of self-directed learning, an on-line medical terminology class, and a comprehensive test one-month after hiring. As another part of the curriculum, new hires work as teaching assistants in EHR training classes. This reinforces their application training and exposes them to typical questions about EHR use.

Team Members

Each of the ten implementation teams includes an advisor (0.2 FTE), analysts (2.0 FTE), a trainer (0.5 FTE), a system administrator (0.2 FTE), and a physician informatician (0.2 FTE). The advisor (an experienced implementation analyst) is responsible for guiding the development of a detailed implementation plan, reviewing the completed analysis, overseeing issue resolution and serving as liaison to the software vendor. The analysts (at least one of them a veteran of other implementations) provide detailed analysis of the practice's workflows, develop practice-specific selection lists (e.g., diagnosis and medication lists), analyze order transmittal needs, recommend new clinical workflows, and provide training and support before and after go-live. The trainers (many of them temporary employees) demonstrate the system to each user, provide multiple brief training sessions to users during the weeks before go-live, and provide in-depth training (eight hours for physicians and support staff) within three days before go-live. The physician informatician is responsible for working through the departmental domain expert (see Chapter 9) to provide practice-specific note templates and order sets, coaching and support for individual physicians, and vetting of new workflows. The program director meets weekly with each implementation team to monitor timelines and address barriers to implementation.

With this team structure in place, we were able to implement 43 practices within 12 months in 2002. The teams performed admirably, with many clinicians singling out the temporary and flexible staff for special praise at the conclusion of rollouts.

Summary

Implementation teams of carefully integrated specialists can function more effectively than smaller teams of generalists. (See Chapter 12 for our similar experience with production support teams.) Keeping these complex teams working effectively requires careful training, written responsibility agreements and frequent formal and informal communication among team leaders.

Reference

1. Ash JS, Stavri PZ, Kuperman GJ. A Consensus Statement on Considerations for a Successful CPOE Implementation. *JAMA* 2003;10:229–234.

Part Two
Support

7
Usability

James M. Walker

EHRs capable of uniting disparate data from many sources are creating the potential for a revolution in the presentation of clinical information to users. For the first time, it is possible (e.g., in the case of a patient with suspected meningitis) to collect information from the chemistry lab, microbiology lab, and radiology department and present the information in formats that are consistent with the needs of the intended users—clinical and administrative workers, and patients.

Constraints

Despite this opportunity, the usability of the EHR characteristically gets short shrift, for many reasons:

- From the perspective of software vendors (and implementation teams), designing for usability requires extra effort:
  "It's really interesting to watch engineers and computer scientists go about designing a product. They argue and argue about how to do things, generally with a sincere desire to do the right thing for the user. But when it comes to assessing the trade-offs between the user interface and internal resources in a product, they almost always tend to simplify their own lives. They will have to do the work. They try to make the internal machine architecture as simple as possible. Design teams really need vocal advocates for the people who will ultimately use the interface" (1).
- EHR implementation teams usually do not include a member trained in usability engineering.
- Healthcare team members (clinical and administrative) are invaluable for assessing the usability of an EHR, but rarely have skills in designing for usability. ("The user is always right, but the user doesn't know what he needs." Jakob Nielsen, leading usability expert)

The Case for Usability

Nevertheless, usability is vital. First, poor usability endangers patients. For example, an FDA study of 400 deaths caused by medication errors found that 16 percent were due to name mix-ups; only the wrong dose was a larger culprit (2).

Second, the usability of an EHR critically affects implementation success. Many of the most common complaints physicians have against EHRs relate to poor usability

(3). Below a certain threshold of usability, the implementation will be endangered. A vivid example of this is the fate of the first go-live of Cedars-Sinai's $31-million EHR project. Doctors refused to use the system saying that "it was endangering patient safety and required too much work" (4). Massaro et al. provide an older but more fully documented example in another organization (5).

Faster Is Better: Efficiency and the Quality of Care

There is a tendency to regard the care process efficiencies that are achievable with an EHR as primarily relating to decreasing costs and increasing provider satisfaction (and use). In this view, improved care quality is achieved in a different way—through such clinical decision support tools as allergy and drug-drug interaction checking and best practice reminders. However, in our experience, and in the experience of companies like Motorola, improving efficiency is among the most powerful means of improving quality: "... one of the fastest ways to improve quality is to focus on reducing cycle time. . . . *[With a focus]* on cycle time, defects were reduced at a much faster rate than *[when focusing]* on defect reduction alone" (6).

There are many reasons for this. The clinical work of physicians and nurses is frequently interrupted, often by matters of little or no clinical significance. (7) (8) (9) Clinical anecdote, the limits of short-term memory (10), and the science of error (11) (12) all indicate that these interruptions have the potential to compromise patient care. Reducing these interruptions through better-integrated workflows should reduce error. Increased efficiency in the management of essentially clerical tasks, such as preventative care checking (e.g., checking whether a patient is due for her mammogram) or remembering the elements of the Mini-Mental Status Exam (MMSE), could also enable clinicians to spend more time on the cognitive and skill-based aspects of patient care, including communicating with patients.

For all these reasons, we regard improved care-process efficiency as a critical first step in improving quality of care. This causal linkage is assumed throughout the book.

The Business Case for Usability

For a CDO, the financial benefits of a more rather than less usable implementation are hard to measure, but can be reasonably estimated. Assume conservatively that a more (rather than less) usable EHR saves each physician 10 minutes a day: 10 minutes a day × 220 days a year × $100 dollars an hour = $3,520 per physician per year (×600 physicians in our system = $2,112,000 a year). Although there is no guarantee that time savings will translate into higher productivity, the steadily increasing pressure on physicians to be more productive makes the translation likely.

For software developers, improved usability also can lead to financial benefit. An IBM study concluded that $1 spent on usability in the design phase results in a $100 internal return (13). Landauer, Karat and Chapanis document the general business case for usability (14–16).

Software Design

Many factors contribute to an EHR's usability. The most fixed is the basic design of the EHR software. While local implementation decisions have a more immediate impact on usability, the fundamental design of the EHR software determines the limits of what those local decisions can accomplish. Gartner's and KLAS's reviews provide access both to consultant assessments (17) and to the aggregated experience of CIOs and senior project managers with various products (18).

Usability testing should be an explicit part of the pre-purchase assessment of EHR software. To achieve this, have the vendor demonstrate how their software can be used to work through clinical scenarios, which represent your primary clinical workflows:

- Find the patient's latest LDL result.
- How many coronary artery disease risk factors does the patient have? What is the patient's risk of having a coronary-disease related event in the next 5 years?
- Schedule the patient for a linked rheumatology visit and injection-room treatment.
- Order lab tests to look for medical causes of depression and print out a patient education handout for the patient.
- Review your plan for managing the patient's hypertension.
- What is the nature of the patient's penicillin allergy?
- Order an orthopaedics consult, with appropriate pre-visit testing.
- Send a letter to the patient reporting on her thyroid test result, order thyroid medicine, and schedule repeat testing for six weeks from now.

As the scenarios play out, ask these questions:

- How easily can the user accomplish the task?
- Is screen space used efficiently?
- Is the screen space well organized?
- Is it easy to find your way around?
- Does the system appear easy to learn?
- Are both beginners and experts accommodated?
- Are extraneous, confusing choices offered?
- Does the EHR make the work easier?
- Does it make the work faster?

Minimizing the number of different EHR applications (e.g., inpatient, outpatient, special-purpose) that clinicians must use is also important. Every additional EHR system increases memory requirements and the likelihood of negative transference, decreasing the likelihood that clinicians will become effective users.

Transference

Transference is the name given to the observation that previously acquired knowledge and skills carry over and affect learning of new information and skills. As example of positive transference, if a new application closes when the user clicks on the small box with an X in it in the upper right hand corner of the screen, that part of the application will not require learning at all. It will seem intuitive, if the user even becomes conscious of it. Using the same labels for the same functions and locating the same function in the same place are two important ways to use the power of positive transference to help EHR users.

On the other hand, if the user must click on a "standard" close box in some settings, a different box, labeled "Close", in other settings, a button labeled "Exit" in other settings, and a box labeled "Exit Workspace" in yet others, the result will be confusion and very hard learning. The confusion will be compounded if the boxes are in different places on different screens.

Many of the principles in this chapter represent methods of maximizing positive transference from clinicians' other knowledge and skills to their learning of the EHR—and minimizing negative transference.

Workflow Redesign

A usable EHR will reflect current workflows or widely-accepted process improvements. Although a failure to introduce process improvements as part of an EHR implementation can result in the perpetuation of suboptimal workflows, implementing radical or controversial changes will increase the difficulty of learning (through negative transference) and will prompt some users to create dysfunctional workarounds (see Chapter 5 for a more extended discussion).

The User Interface

The user interface must use clear design to provide easy access to complex information. A key element of clarity is designing the interface of the EHR to reflect standard clinical workflows (19). For example, the movement of thought from eliciting the patient's presenting problem (or chief complaint) through the history, review of systems, physical examination, assessment, and plan provides a simple outline that can be used to organize the complexities of most patient encounters. Similarly, inpatient orders consistently follow this flow: Admit to __ (unit), Diagnosis, Condition, Vitals, Allergies, Nursing Orders, Drugs (Specific and Symptomatic), and Labs (and other tests). This order provides a powerful framework for presenting order sets and for streamlining clinicians' review of active orders. Nursing assessments, clinical guidelines, care pathways, and discharge documents also provide built-in opportunities to structure the appearance and navigation of the EHR interface in ways that make the EHR appear intuitive to users.

Simplicity is at the heart of clarity. According to Jakob Nielsen, "Simplicity may be the single most important usability guideline. The less stuff you show users, the less they'll have to scan and comprehend, and the better the odds that they'll pick the correct option at any given stage. Duplicating features adds significant overhead to both the scanning process and the comprehension process" (20). This is due, in large part, to the fact that the capacity of short-term memory is fixed at a maximum of nine elements, has a maximum duration of 15 seconds (unless refreshed), and is easily disturbed by interruptions. Thus, while the interface must provide access to a wealth of patient-specific and general medical information a click or two away, it must also be designed to help clinicians focus rapidly on the most relevant information.

Recognition, Not Memory

One way to save short-term memory for critical tasks is to allow users to substitute recognition for memory whenever possible. For example, a button labeled "Results" requires only recognition, while clicking F6 to review results requires memory and is, therefore, harder to perform (10) (19). Of course, some actions will be performed so many times by at least some users that memory will be efficient (e.g., clicking F2 to move through each element of a note template). This efficiency declines rapidly as the number of actions to be remembered increases and their frequency of use declines.

Layered Lists

A key advantage of electronic medical records over paper is the ability of the EHR to provide users simplified lists of options, with extended lists (often including hundreds of options) a single click away. A reasonable rule of thumb is to include the four to eight most frequently used selections in the concise list, listed in order of frequency. The remainder of the list should be alphabetized, for efficient searching. This produces lists that fit most user's needs rapidly and require scrolling (which decreases reading speed (21)) only infrequently. The careful selection of list components also presents an opportunity to support optimal practice. Include only preferred interventions (tests, treatments, referrals, patient education materials) in the concise lists (making the right thing easier to do), while other interventions that may be appropriate less frequently remain available in the more comprehensive lists.

A particularly powerful method of simplification relates to the input of clinical observations. Clinicians routinely record data which does not aid in distinguishing one diagnosis from another simply because it is not humanly possible to remember whether the data is relevant to a given problem. At the same time (and for the same reason), data that does distinguish one diagnosis from another is frequently not documented. Using note templates, the EHR can provide users with a rapid means of documenting, for example, the 16 criteria that distinguish benign low-back pain from pain that warrants emergency MRI and X-ray therapy (22). (If you are a generalist physician, see how many of the sixteen you can jot down before checking the list in Appendix 6.)

Memory prompts and facilitated documentation of relevant clinical observations (both positive and negative) produce clinically relevant collections of information—and can do so in less time than it takes to write or dictate. For example, the typical back pain examination (in which all sixteen of Deyo's diagnostic criteria are negative) can be recorded in seven mouse clicks (See Figure 15.1). These precision data sets are harder to create than are "complete" lists of signs and symptoms—which some EHR vendors pay medical students to compile—but are markedly more usable (and clinically pertinent).

EHR Behavior: Hard or Soft Stops

A hard stop is a software feature that prevents the user from going on until he performs a required action (e.g., entering a billing code before closing an office visit note). A soft stop requires only that the user acknowledge a recommendation, typically with a single mouse click, before going on.

Some EHR developers and operations managers favor using hard stops to force clinicians to use the EHR as intended. As Walker's Fourth Law of Informatics puts it: "Everyone wants to use the EHR to make someone else do something." This is, at least in part, because computer professionals and managers ". . . tend to place high value on efficiency and predictability, and to devalue the need for human discretion and innovation" (23). This leads them to underestimate the difficulty of creating rules which are so comprehensively appropriate that they must be followed in every situation (the necessary prerequisite for a hard stop). Because healthcare is profoundly complex, universally applicable rules will be few and far between (24). Worse, patient care is often highly time-sensitive and hard stops have the potential to cause serious patient harm, particularly by confusing or delaying ordering. Perhaps fortunately, users are remarkably skillful at creating (and sharing) workarounds that subvert the intention of hard stops. Rather than hard stops, we prefer to provide a real-time reminder of best practice, an order set for putting the recommendation into action, and a place for the physician to document his reasoning if the recommendation is dismissed. Finally, we create physician-specific performance reports that are automatically generated and transmitted to the appropriate manager for review and any necessary action.

Information Display

Healthcare information is produced by laboratory personnel (test results and interpretations), radiology personnel (images and their interpretation), and other clinicians. Clinicians, patients, and various administrative personnel are consumers of that information. Producers and consumers have different approaches to information. Information producers think in terms of the means of production ("Was the stress test performed with thallium or cardiolyte?") and the means that support its production ("Is the test performed in the chemistry lab or the hematology lab?"). While this perspective is appropriate for information producers, it does not focus on the primary concerns of information consumers and does not lead to usable informational display.

An information consumer may access a specific clinical datum (e.g., a lab test result) anywhere from daily to a few times a year. They order many tests performed by different information producers that focus on answering a specific clinical question, for example an India ink, Gram stain, CSF analysis, and CT scan to answer the question whether a patient has meningitis. Their preferred organization of the tests is based on the question asked, not the details of the test's performance. They access the information in multiple contexts, some of which provide added information (e.g., a glucose measurement in patient with neuroglycopenic symptoms) and some that provide little information (e.g., a normal random glucose performed six months ago). Clinicians may act on test results in time-pressured settings, frequently accompanied by interruptions (9). This makes maximum readability and minimal ambiguity in clinical information displays critical.

EHRs often limit the number of characters available for display names. And although it would be possible for EHR developers to enable various users—information-tion producers and consumers alike—to see their own preferred form of the name, many EHRs do not provide this feature, requiring that all users see the same name. This means that implementation teams must negotiate with information producers to find names that are acceptable for multiple audiences—clinical and administrative. (See box.)

A Rose by Any Other Name

"LD" has become the standard name for lactate dehydrogenase in clinical chemistry (25) (26), while "LDH" remains standard usage among physicians. When our lab changed the name in the laboratory information system to "LD," the change was transferred to the EHR, and physicians who typed "LDH" found themselves unable to find the test. We created "LDH" as a synonym for "LD," so that users can find "LD" by typing "LDH." (Of course, this does not solve the problem that the test result is displayed as "LD," doubtless costing many clinicians a moment to recall that "LDH" is called "LD" by the lab.)

Principles and Conventions

Much of our knowledge regarding optimal clinical information presentation must be extrapolated from other settings, and generalizability is problematic. Empirical studies in healthcare are few and methodologically weak. The principles that follow are supported by expert opinion and/or by feedback sessions conducted with over 100 physicians, mid-level providers, nurses, and laboratory staff. The references are to particularly well-reasoned or documented articles.

First Principle: Every principle and convention is subservient to the goal of rapid, unambiguous communication.

Organization

1. Organize test results by clinical relationships, not by source.
   a. Some clusters of tests are so fixed in the minds of clinicians that there is no advantage in "optimizing" their contents (e.g., electrolytes and blood counts).
   b. Some tests may be grouped together without conflicting with established thought patterns:
      - Tests of cerebrospinal fluid.
      - Diabetes-HbA1c, glucose, microalbumin, LDL.
      - Lipid panel, ALT, CK.

2. Present the most commonly ordered and referred to tests first (e.g., electrolytes, renal, CBC, hepatic function).
3. Group tests according to their most common use:
   a. Levels of drugs that have a significant therapeutic use are displayed in "Drug Monitoring".
   b. Levels of drugs that have limited or no therapeutic use are displayed in "Toxicology."
5. Arrange displays consistently, avoiding the need to use conscious thought for navigation.
6. Organize data:
   a. Likely to require conscious thought in tables (e.g., serum digoxin level).
   b. Likely to be significant primarily as a constituent of a pattern (e.g., a ventilator rate from 48 hours previous) as part of a graphic (27). See Figure 7.1.
7. Since humans can process only five to nine items at a time, arranging items into meaningful constellations of (e.g., lipid panel, ALT, CK) data improves performance: (28)
   a. Use proximity to link related data.
   b. Use white space to separate unrelated data and to increase readability.
8. Avoid the need for scrolling, which disorients users and delays location of pertinent information.

Presenting Words

1. "Jargon is fine—the user's jargon not yours." Jakob Nielsen (19).
2. Avoid the use of words spelled entirely in capital letters. Skilled readers read the shapes of words or even phrases as wholes, rather than reading individual letters. (Whether or not "Tall Man" letters will aid clinicians in selecting the right drug in an EHR does not appear to have been studied, but is a question worth considering. See www.fda.gov/cder/drug/mederrors/namediff.htm.)
3. Serif fonts make blocks of text (as opposed to headlines) more readable (29).
4. The most important part of the label should appear first and most prominently (e.g., **Neut, abs** rather than **Abs neut**).
5. If the spaces between the words of a label must be eliminated (a common need due to software limitations), place lower case letters immediately next to upper case letters (e.g., **FibrinogenNK**). But beware of the potentially confusing effect of removing spaces.
6. Space flexibly when it is necessary to shorten a label or influence the alphabetical order of lists:
   a. Remove the space after a comma (e.g., **Xylose, bld**).
   b. Remove the space between most symbols and the word that follows (e.g., **#Counted**).
7. Mimic oral usage
   a. The label should read like the spoken form of the test name (e.g., **Thiocyan** versus **Thio CN**).
   b. The display name should *begin* as much like the spoken form of the test as possible (e.g., **Ethylene gly** instead of **Eth glycol**).
8. To avoid redundancy, minimize the use of the following terms in display names
   a. Titer.
   b. Ratio.

c. "Quantitative"—unless there is a qualitative form

d. Blood, serum, and plasma are assumed, unless they are needed to distinguish among tests.

9. Abbreviations and Acronyms

a. Use the briefest, most easily recognized form of the name, e.g., **K**, **BUN**, **Cr**, **Alb**.

c. Three-letter abbreviations and acronyms provide an optimal balance of brevity and clarity (30). For example, PE and PT have multiple possible meanings, while DVT and TIA are unmistakable.

d. Use all capital letters for acronyms (e.g., ASA) and mixed case for abbreviations (e.g., Mag).

e. Avoid ambiguous abbreviations, for example,
    i. Comm (for comment).
    ii. Cyst (for cystine).

f. Avoid dangerous abbreviations. (For a minimum list see "Prohibited Abbreviations—See Goal 2" at www.jcaho.org.)

10. Parentheses

a. Use parentheses to de-emphasize the elements of names that are of secondary importance, but necessary. For example, "CRP (hs)" for high-sensitivity C-reactive protein.

b. Discard parentheses when necessary to shorten names.

11. Label only nuclear medicine studies as "scans."

Case: Create Unambiguous Prescriptions

CORTISPORIN OT: 3 GTT QD
CORTISPORIN OP: 1 GTT OU QD

These names for two different formulations of the medicine Cortisporin are similar enough that, although a physician ordered OP (for ophthalmic, intended to be used in the eye), the pharmacist misread the (computer-printed!) prescription and dispensed OT (for otic, intended for use in the ear) with instructions for application to the eye. (Note how the EHR-required all-capitals display contributes to the similarity of the names and administration instructions.)

To reduce the risk of a recurrence, we renamed the formulations to create maximum contrast among them. The dispensing information was translated into standard English to further decrease the risk of a pharmacist or patient misunderstanding the medication's intended use. Because even some specialists are unclear regarding which formulation to use for eardrum perforations, we added that indication to the appropriate formulation.

CORTISPORIN OTIC SUSP (FOR PERFORATION): 4 DROPS IN AFFECTED EAR DAILY
CORTISPORIN OTIC SOLN: 4 DROPS IN AFFECTED EAR DAILY
CORTISPORIN OPHTHALMIC SOLN: 2 DROPS IN AFFECTED EYE DAILY
CORTISPORIN OPHTHALMIC OINTMENT: 1/4-INCH IN AFFECTED EYE DAILY

Color

One of the primary challenges in displaying test results is to streamline the tedious and error-prone task of identifying the relatively few abnormal results among the hundreds of results that are often available for a patient. The skillful use of color can make this task dramatically easier and less error-prone.

1. The most visible color to most humans is "optic yellow" (31). This is the color of tennis balls, newer fire trucks, highway signs, and police cordon tape.
2. Blue (particularly a medium 'Internet' blue) is the color most easily distinguished from other colors (32).
3. Black text on white background is the easiest to read.
4. Black text on an optic yellow background combines maximum visibility with high readability.
5. Humans are least sensitive to red (31). To make a design element recede into the background, color it red. (In highway signs and lights and Internet browsers, red means stop.)

Case: Highlight Abnormal Test Results

Putting a yellow background behind abnormal results makes them instantly visible. The use of Internet blue for new results and black for results that have already been viewed makes it easy to focus on new results. Both the blue and black are easily read on the yellow background. (See Figure 7.1.)

Numbers

1. Numbers are most readable in tables. In one small study, tables were at least as quickly and accurately read as icons (graphics), text, or pie charts by both physicians and nurses. (33) "Tables usually outperform graphics in reporting on small data sets of 20 numbers or less. The special power of graphics comes in the display of large data sets" (32). For this reason, graphical displays of information are more likely to be useful in intensive-care units than in other settings (34). (See Figure 7.2.)

2. Display numbers in rows rather than columns. All but one of 120 feedback participants preferred repetitive test results (e.g., temperatures, potassium readings) to be displayed in horizontal rows. (See Figure 7.1.)

3. Round numbers to two significant digits. There is experimental evidence that any interruption reduces the capacity of short-term memory to two digits. The loss of accuracy due to rounding to two significant digits has been calculated to be 3.4%, well within acceptable limits for clinical decision-making (35). For example, clinical decision-making will not change if a TSH is reported as 2.4 rather than 2.37 or 2.43. For a few tests whose results are three-digit integers (e.g. serum sodium) the third digit is clinically relevant.

These numbers would be
Internet blue because they are
unreviewed results.

The cells which are
highlighted gray would be
highlighted yellow on screen.

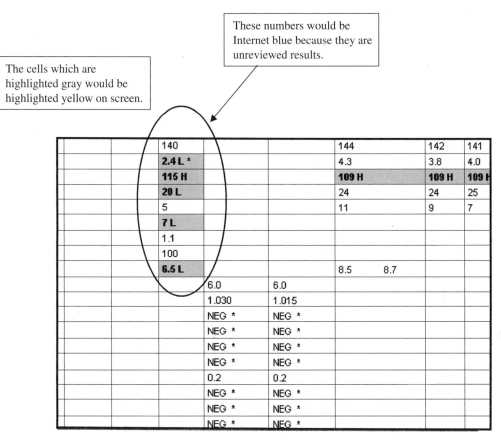

FIGURE 7.1. Use of Color to Highlight New and Abnormal Results.

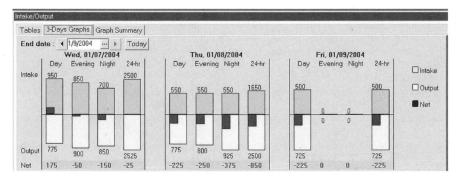

FIGURE 7.2. Graphical Display of Complex Data. (Copyright © 2000–2004 Epic Systems Corporation).

Usability Testing

Although a usability testing lab is ideal, you do not need one to refine the usability of your EHR system build. Give as few as four typical users (both sophisticated and naïve) clinical tasks in scripted scenarios. Ask them to think out loud as they work through the tasks using the EHR. Four users are enough to identify 80% of interface problems (36). If feasible, representatives of the implementation team and the training team should observe this testing. An observation room with one-way glass is helpful but not required (37).

Summary

Although creating a usable EHR requires careful attention, it is fundamentally a matter of learning from usable and unusable software interfaces and applying a fairly simple set of design and testing principles to your purchase and customization of the EHR.

References

1. King M. A telephone company designer, commenting on an early draft of POET, quoted in Norman D. *The Psychology of Everyday Things*. Basic Books; 1998, p.156.
2. Neergaard L. Labels on Drugs to Battle Mix-Ups. Chicago: *Tribune*; January 1, 2002.
3. Rousseau N, McColl E, Newton J, Grimshaw J, Eccles M. Practice based, longitudinal, qualitative interview study of computerised evidence based guidelines in primary care. *Br Med J* 2003;326:314.
4. Ornstein C. Hospital Heeds Doctors, Suspends Use of Software. Los Angeles: *Times*, January 22, 2003.
5. Massaro T. Introducing physician order entry at a major academic medical center: I. Impact on organizational culture and behavior. *Acad Med* 1993;68:20–25.
6. Schmidt WH, Finnigan JP. *The Race Without a Finish Line: America's Quest for Total Quality*. San Francisco: Jossey-Bass; 1992.
7. Katz M, Schroeder S. The sounds of the hospital: paging patterns in three teaching hospitals. *New Engl J Med* 1988;319:1585.
8. Blum N, Lieu T. Interrupted care: the effects of paging on pediatric resident activities. *Am J Dis Child* 1992;146:806.
9. Coiera E, Tombs V. Communication behaviours in a hospital setting—an observational study. *Br Med J* 1998;316:673.
10. Boralv E. Usability and efficiency. The HELIOS approach to development of user interfaces. *Comput Methods Programs Biomed* 1994;45(Suppl):S47–64.
11. Reason J. *Human Error*. Cambridge: Cambridge University Press; 1990.
12. Leape L. Learning from Errors. Translating Evidence into Practice; Washington, D.C.: AHCPR; 1997.
13. Zhang. Usability Problems with the electronic medical record. AMIA Fall Conference; Washington, DC: AMIA; 1999.
14. Landauer T. *The Trouble with Computers: Usefulness, Usability, and Productivity*. Cambridge, MA: MIT Press; 1995.
15. Karat C-M. A business case approach to usability. In: Bias R, Mayhew D, editors. *Cost-Justifying Usability*. New York: Academic Press; 1994;45–70.
16. Chapanis A. The business case for human factors in informatics. In: Shackel, Brian, Richardson, editors. *Human Factors for Informatics Usability*. Cambridge: Cambridge University; 1991;39–71.

17. Handler T. *Enterprise CPR Magic Quadrant.* Gartner; 2002.
18. KLAS. CPOE Perception Report 2003.
19. Nielsen J. Ten Usability Heuristics; 1994. www.useit.com/papers/heurestic/heurestic-list.htm
20. Nielsen J. Reduce Redundancy; 2002. www.altimawebsystems.com/resources/articles.shtml?nid+3&cid+26&lid+3
21. Nygren E, Johnson M, Henriksson P. Reading the medical record. II. Design of a human-computer interface for basic reading of computerized medical records. *Comput Methods Programs Biomed* 1992;39:13–25.
22. Deyo, R. (1992). Lower back pain; an update. *American College of Physicians.* San Diego, American College of Physicians: Tape 1-J.
23. Winograd T, Flores F. *Understanding computers and cognition: a new foundation for design.* Reading, MA: Addison-Wesley; 1986.
24. Sittig D. Computer-based order entry: the state of the art. *J Am Med Informatics Assoc* 1994;1:108.
25. Burtis C, Ashwood E, editors. *Tietz Textbook of Clinical Chemistry.* 2nd ed. Philadelphia: W.B. Saunders Company; 1994.
26. IUB Nomenclature Committee. Enzyme Nomenclature, 1978: Recommendations of the Nomenclature Committee of IUB on the Nomenclature and Classification of Enzymes. New York: Academic Press; 1979.
27. Tan, J.K. Health graphics: reconciling theory and practice in the 21st century. *Medinfo*; 1995;8(PT1):796–800.
28. Shneiderman, B. *Designing the User Interface: Strategies for Effective Human-Computer Interaction.* Reading, MA: Addison-Wesley; 1998.
29. Marcus A. *Graphic Design for Electronic Documents and User Interfaces.* New York: ACM Press; 1992.
30. Euzéby JP. Three-letter code for abbreviations of generic names. 2002. www.bacterio.cict.fr/abbreviations.html
31. Cole W. Information Design in Health Care: 19th Annual Symposium on Computer Applications in Medical Care; 1995, New Orleans: AMIA; 1995.
32. Tufte ER. *The Visual Display of Quantitative Information.* Cheshire, Conn: Graphics Press; 1983.
33. Elting L, Bodey G. Is a picture worth a thousand medical words? A randomized trial of reporting formats for medical research data. *Methods of Information in Medicine* 1991;30: 145.
34. Powsner S, Tufte E. Graphical summary of patient status. *Lancet* 1994;344:386.
35. Ehrenberg A. Rudiments of numeracy. *Journal of the Royal Statistical Society* 1977;140: 277–97.
36. Patel V. Interface Design for Health Care Environments: The Role of Cognitive Science. AMIA Fall Symposium. Orlando, FL: AMIA; 1998.
37. Elkin PL, Sorensen B, Palo DD. Optimization of a Research Web Environment for Academic Internal Medicine Faculty. *J Am Med Informatics* 2002;9:472.

Additional Reading

Norman, D. A. (1988). *The Psychology of Everyday Things.* New York: Basic Books.
Highly readable, evocative. The place to start.
Horton, W. (1994). *Designing and Writing Online Documentation.* New York: Wiley.
Masterful and practical. Covers every aspect of designing computer documents.
Nielsen, J. (1993). *Usability Engineering.* Boston, MA: AP Professional.
A highly regarded handbook of computer usability.

8
Training

Wanda L. Krum and Jack D. Latshaw

> *Learning is what most adults will do for a living in the 21st century.*
>
> —*Bob Perelman*

After devoting months to developing a new EHR and improved workflows, your organization will need a wide range of clinical and administrative workers to become skilled users of the EHR suite of applications. Although often under-budgeted (1), training is critical to achieving this goal. Effective training helps users achieve the efficiency and care quality benefits of an EHR. It improves morale and decreases employee turnover. Finally, it communicates your organization's commitment to implementing an effective EHR.

This chapter details methods for developing an effective training program. It will help you understand the characteristics of your audiences, develop effective curricula, identify optimal training strategies and delivery systems, and plan for facility needs.

Adult Learners

Adults are effective learners, in large part because they are critical. They expect training to be meaningful and relevant to their perceived needs. They often ask, "Why do I need to know this?" or "How will I use this?" Effective training must address these questions explicitly and persuasively. Simply showing the user how to use software features is not enough. Most learners are not interested in computers. They are interested in getting their work done faster and easier with no loss of quality. They bring extensive knowledge and experience to the classroom and expect to relate this knowledge to their new learning. For all these reasons, scenarios taken from actual practice are particularly powerful teaching tools.

Adult learners measure their learning by competencies gained, not by seat-time. For them, seat-time is a measure of cost rather than of quality or accomplishment. Learners who already have EHR knowledge or skills or who can learn them on their own will rightly criticize a training system that does not allow them to demonstrate their competency and resume their work. Competency-based training offers CDOs the benefits of decreased employee time spent in training and increased trainer time available for those who really need it.

Self-Paced Learning

Self-paced learning is effective for adult learners and efficient for both the learner and the organization. Nevertheless, on the few occasions when we have tried pilots of self-directed learning as the sole EHR training method for clinicians, we have had to provide emergency trainer-led courses to get users trained in time to meet go-live schedules. In 2004, we installed a computerized learning management system, which promises to make self-paced learning more feasible. We anticipate that its automated reporting capability may make it possible to allow learners who demonstrate competency on all the required training modules of the inpatient EHR by two weeks before go-live to opt out of face-to-face instruction.

Needs Analysis

The first step in creating a training curriculum is to identify the training needs of the practice as the implementation team begins planning the implementation. Participation in team meetings helps trainers to identify these needs. In addition, the team customizes several variables according to practice need and preferences:

- *What are the best times for training?* Typical best times include early morning, lunchtime, and late afternoon (post-clinic) sessions.
- *Should various caregiver types (e.g., physicians, other clinicians, administrative workers) be trained together or separately?* Physicians find it wasteful to attend sessions that include nursing and clerical workflows. Separate training enables learners to benefit from more focused attention to their workflows. To the extent that practice schedules allow it, we provide specific training for providers, nursing personnel, and administrative workers.
- *What are appropriate training scenarios (and other content)?*
- *Who may need special help with training?*
- *Shall the practice reduce the number of patients on provider schedules and for how long?* Most practices reduce scheduled patient volume by 50% the first week and by 25% the next two weeks. However, several of our practices did not reduce appointment schedules at all and did very well. All practices continued to see acute patients as needed.

Training Trainers

A core group of trainers and support staff create training courses and train other trainers (as well as most users). Trainers are enlisted from among trainers currently active elsewhere in the organization and from among interested clinical employees. Each group has characteristic strengths and weaknesses. Currently active trainers may need to learn clinical workflows and medical terminology. (To help them understand learners' work and language, we have them provide shadowing support in practices that are going live. We also require an on-line course that reviews general and specialty-specific clinical terminology.) Clinical employees know the workflows and terminology and appreciate the potential of the EHR to improve healthcare processes, but may need to learn training skills. On the whole, we find it easier to teach interested clinicians training skills than to teach trainers clinical workflows and language.

All trainers go through a process of credentialing, which includes demonstrating the following competencies:

1. Demonstrating the EHR to users
2. Training each phase of the EHR in the presence of a credentialed trainer
3. When time constraints preclude numbers 1 and 2, trainers are required to take a test to demonstrate their understanding of the EHR.

New trainers usually strengthen their understanding of the EHR by participating in training classes conducted by an experienced trainer and by providing shadowing support to new users. In large classes, new trainers help learners who need extra attention. This allows the new trainer to work in a supervised setting and the lead trainer to teach at a pace appropriate to the majority of the students. Implementation analysts also work in this training support role to prepare them for their work on the production support team.

Pre Go-Live Training

To be effective, training needs to be given just in time, a week (or at most two) before go-live. Training intensifies at go-live and needs to be readily available as long as the EHR is in use.

The great impediments to just-in-time training are its added complexity and cost. Rather than scheduling a few four-hour classroom sessions over several weeks, the training team will need to schedule many 45-minute sessions within a week or two of go-live. (Rather than considering training complete a few weeks after go-live, the team will need to find cost-effective methods to answer user questions and provide ongoing EHR training over several years.)

In the week or two before go-live, users need to learn just enough to get them through the tasks that comprise the bulk of their work. A 45-minute session is near the limit of sustainable concentration on new material. Many users (particularly physicians and nurses) are unlikely to be available for more than 90 minutes of face-to-face instruction during any two-week period. This mandates a concentrated focus on the knowledge and skills each type of user needs in order to use the EHR effectively. It also makes online instruction an important adjunct.

Go-Live Shadowing

The next stage of training is provided by trainers who shadow users during go-live. This shadowing gives new users rapid answers to their questions as they start to use the EHR in their work. It also gives trainers the opportunity to identify gaps in users' skills and provide focused training to close the gaps. We make shadowing available to every user during all working hours for the first two weeks of go-live.

Post-implementation Training

As shadowing support ends, users direct their questions to the Help Desk, who answer basic questions (first and second shift) and triage advanced questions to the trainer on call for the production-support team. During the first three months of 2003, with 43 clinics in their first year of implementation and 3,850 active users, the production support team answered over 1,200 questions.

The post implementation review, scheduled about one month after go-live, provides the first formal assessment of the practice's ongoing training needs and initiates the post-implementation training program. This review is critical to implementation effectiveness, but can fall prey to implementation resource conflicts. To minimize those conflicts, we have moved this function to a team that reports to clinical leadership, while still coordinating its activities closely with the EHR implementation team.

Remote Training

On-call availability is essential to most IT support systems. We have adapted this model to provide ongoing just-in-time EHR training with a "Trainer On Call." When an EHR question is outside the Help Desk's scope, they transfer the caller to a production-support analyst who is the Trainer On Call. This trainer can use software to see and control the caller's computer remotely. Both the user and the trainer can see the screen and both can use the keyboard and mouse to work through the problem. Because instructors are able to see the user's computer screen, they can understand the caller's question clearly and show the caller exactly how to use the software. This individualized, just-in-time instruction saves the user time, increases learning and makes efficient use of EHR team resources. It combines a rapid response to a pressing user need (the "teachable moment") with audiovisual support that makes learning memorable. It produces great user satisfaction. Because of its effectiveness, we have begun to use classes conducted by the Trainer On Call as a replacement for face-to-face instruction—primarily when individual learners would otherwise have to travel hours to a classroom.

Trainers On Call need several competencies: First, they must be able to use the multitasking capabilities of Windows® effectively. Microsoft Office User Specialist certification is a useful measure of this competency. The second competency is in-depth knowledge of how the EHR suite of applications is used in practice. This competency is acquired through a combination of formal classes, experience in classroom teaching, shadow training and answering Help Desk calls. The third competency is the ability to empathize with callers and avoid taking personally any frustration they may express.

Users' Group Meetings

An annual users' group meeting (UGM) can be an effective means of promoting increased efficiency of EHR use, celebrating implementation milestones, and publicizing upcoming projects. All clinical and administrative EHR users are invited. Morning plenary sessions focus on issues of broad interest, while afternoon breakout sessions focus on the interests of specific groups. Among our most popular offerings are the "Tips and Tricks" classes and the "Talk-Back" sessions with the senior EHR Project Manager and the Chief Medical Information Officer. As with any such meeting, the opportunity to share insights with other users is one of the major benefits of the day. To encourage this, we schedule plenty of time for informal discussion, particularly at lunch. Providing continuing professional education credits encourages participation.

We staff the UGM with EHR team members and with clinical and administrative EHR users with excellent communications skills. Ninety-seven percent of users rate the day as a very good or excellent learning experience (4 or 5 on a 5-point Likert scale). Since its inception, UGM attendance has increased each year.

Upgrade Training

Minor software upgrades necessitate little training and no classroom instruction. Major upgrades require more learning, although managers and users are loath to spend more than a single 45-minute session on face-to-face training. Our training methodology is the same as for initial implementations. We provide super-users a more comprehensive trainer-led session to prepare them to support other members of their practices.

New Hires

Initially, the need to train new staff physicians, residents, students, and other new EHR users was small. We provided one-on-one training on demand. As the need grew, we shifted to offering trainer-led classes once a month on the main campus. Since access to the EHR is not granted until training is complete, a delay in training means a loss of productivity. Thus, managers have requested more frequent training sessions. We now offer two one-day, five-hour classes every week at each hospital. One day is designed for providers and the second for non-providers. Training continues to be scenario-based, but since the participants are no longer from the same practice, training follows generic workflows. Users learn practice-specific workflows in their practice, usually from their super-user.

Site managers may request one day of shadowing support for new providers after they have completed training. This is an adequate supplement to the initial training for most users. In fact, most new users prefer to get post-training support from fellow workers, particularly from super-users. (Super-users are selected by practice managers for their leadership abilities, interpersonal skills, understanding of the practice's workflows, enthusiasm, and ability to incorporate new or changing software into their work. They commit themselves to learn and apply new EHR functions to their work and to provide support to the other members of their practices.)

The online curriculum discussed below enables users to do self-paced learning on advanced features or topics they missed during the trainer-led class.

Training Housestaff and Medical Students

The arrangements for new hires are not adequate for housestaff (residents and fellows), due to the large cohort that requires training every July. They need full EHR training, but classroom training is inadequate and unnecessary in view of their general comfort with computers and previous exposure to EHRs. Medical and other health-care students need efficient training even more, since they cycle through rotations every two to six weeks. Fortunately, they only need to learn a limited set of EHR functions.

Responding to this set of needs, a team of educators and EHR staff developed an online training course for housestaff and students (which has turned out to be useful to other new employees). An instructional designer from the education office worked with two members of the EHR team to develop content to meet specific learning objectives. The objectives introduce each module and determine the content of the post-tests. The designer chose instructional strategies that allow learners to set their own pace—entering, exiting, reviewing, and skipping over modules as needed. Simple presentation technologies kept development time and costs down.

The course has been well received by housestaff and students, who no longer need extensive training from staff physicians. Its use as an adjunct to classroom sessions has been extended to all new hires.

The Software Training Environment

If training is conducted in the production environment of the EHR, both the integrity of the database and patient confidentiality will be at risk. Early in the implementation, one learner was observed clicking the e-signature button, unaware that he was electronically signing all his notes without reviewing them. To avoid this risk, we created a training environment that mirrors the production EHR environment. The training environment gives users a safe place to learn by trial and error. It also gives trainers a controlled setting in which practice patients and scenarios can be created and then refreshed for successive groups of learners.

While it is effective, the use of a training environment has its costs. Keeping the training environment synchronized with the production environment requires a technical team member's skills. However, we have never assigned a technical team member to be responsible for the training environment. As a result, synchronization of the training environment with the production environment has a low priority and is usually done only at the specific request of the training team.

In our EHR product, practice-specific documentation tools (e.g., note templates and order sets) must be built in both environments for each practice's implementation. The resources needed to create these multiple instances are often unavailable. If the trainers have time, they build a sample set of documentation tools. If not, they use a generic documentation tool to illustrate the functions the user will need to know.

In spite of the complexity of building and maintaining it, the training environment's realism and safety makes it the preferred setting for training. The exception to this is teaching read-only activities, such as results review, although even in that case, it is important to remind students to view only the records of their own patients.

Training Wheels

Most practices have no space for a temporary training room, and many of our clinicians would lose a full day of work travelling back and forth for training on one of our hospital campuses. For us, the solution to these constraints is a mobile computer classroom (Figure 8.1). "Training Wheels" is a van that contains space and computer equipment for six students and a trainer, along with a generator for power. The computers can connect to the network at any Geisinger site. The trainers drive the truck and can prepare it for a class in 15 minutes.

Training wheels was so well received for training at remote sites that we now use it to expand our classroom capacity at the hospitals during peak training periods.

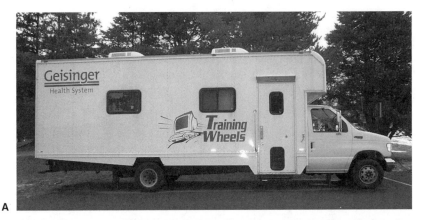

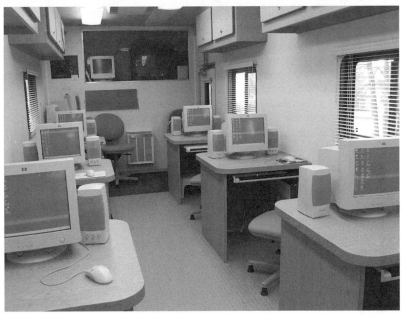

FIGURE 8.1. (A) Training wheels truck. (B) View from the back of the classroom. Notice the windows to help relieve the feeling of being in a small space and the storage cabinets overhead.

Summary

Training clinicians to use an EHR is a complex task, which is critical to the success of the EHR project and the future of the CDO. It requires close attention to the learning characteristics and needs of clinicians; a deep understanding of the EHR and clinical workflows; and flexible methods and content.

Reference

1. Degoulet P, Fieschi M. *Introduction to Clinical Informatics.* New York: Springer; 1997.

9
Clinical Decision Support

JAMES M. WALKER and STEPHEN T. TINGLEY

A man is driving home on a rainy night. He notices a small amber light has appeared on the dashboard in the shape of a gas pump. At the next exit, he pulls over, finds a gas station, and fills the tank.

This scenario is so familiar that it is almost invisible to us, but it provides an example of effective decision support. In this case, several things did and did not happen. What did not happen? The signal did not stop the car from running until gas was added. It did not try to teach the driver something new, nor did it try to convince the driver to do something with which he disagreed.

What did happen? The light provided a non-intrusive alert that helped the driver avoid an unpleasant outcome. The car was programmed to turn on the amber light (whose color was chosen carefully for its visibility) when the fuel tank neared empty. The driver recognized the signal as a prompt to buy gas—without having to refer to his owner's manual. The light came on while there was still time to find gas.

This chapter discusses how to design your EHR build to provide clinical decision support (CDS) as effectively as your car does. We assume that most CDOs will soon conclude that accreditation, care-quality, and reimbursement all require them to implement effective CDS in an EHR. This assumption is based on a research literature that provides good evidence of the efficacy of small numbers of CDS interventions in research settings using non-commercial EHRs. (See Bates, et al. for a recent review (1).) The assumption is also based on the anecdotal experience of thousands of EHR users, who find the prospect of practicing without CDS—for instance, allergy and drug-drug interaction checking—simply frightening. Finally, the assumption is based on the concerted movement of payers and regulators to require, and perhaps even pay for, provider and hospital performance that is not feasible without EHR-based CDS.

Definition

For the purposes of this book, we define CDS as any EHR-related process that gives a clinician patient-related healthcare information with the intent of making the clinician's decision-making more efficient and better informed. While giving patients clinical decision support is vital, it is largely beyond the scope of current EHRs. (See

Chapter 19 for a discussion of our first steps toward the use of the EHR to provide CDS to patients.)

The Need for CDS

Why do we need CDS? Are not clinicians intelligent, committed, and efficient users of information? Certainly, this is true. It is also true that we are human, performing complex intellectual tasks under stringent time constraints and with frequent interruptions. For these reasons, we fall prey to many of the causes of human error, particularly to the limitations of working memory. A recent report documenting pervasive error in American healthcare can be found in McGlynn et al. (2).

Consider this typical example: A 52 year-old woman with diabetes and a history of heart attack two years ago comes to her doctor's office. The patient reports that she would like a routine check-up, but also notes a week of ankle pain. In the 15 to 20 minutes the physician has with this patient, the physician must consider many questions: Has the patient had a recent Pap test, mammogram, and colorectal cancer screening? When was her latest hemoglobin A1C and what was the result? Is it flu season and, if so, does she need vaccination? Does the practice have any more doses of vaccine available? What is her pneumococcal vaccine status? Has she had eye and foot exams within the last year? What is the patient's cholesterol status and blood pressure control? What are appropriate targets for this patient and her actual risk if she doesn't meet them? Is the patient taking appropriate medicines to protect her heart and kidneys? Has she had her urine checked for protein in the last year? Has she had any symptoms of low blood sugar? What is her risk of having osteoporosis? Is she taking calcium and Vitamin D in appropriate doses to prevent it? Has she been tested? Has she had any recent symptoms that might indicate worsening heart disease? Oh, and by the way, what's causing that ankle pain?

Most of the questions raised in this example are fairly straightforward. Providers would generally agree with their clinical importance. The difficulty is in remembering all of the questions, finding the information needed (both patient-specific and general) to answer each one, and negotiating a plan for each one with the patient—along with diagnosing and treating the ankle pain. Yarnall, et al, estimate that it would take a physician seven hours each working day to implement the United States Preventive Services Task Force disease-prevention guidelines (3). If the EHR can be programmed to help clinicians and patients identify and answer these questions efficiently, it will produce remarkable improvements in care quality and patient outcomes.

Types of CDS

Although CDS interventions are often divided into active alerts and passive reminders, the situation is not so simple. As Table 9.1 illustrates, CDS interventions can be characterized in at least two dimensions. On one axis reminders range from intrusive reminders that obscure the screen to non-intrusive reminders that make information available but do not interrupt the user's work. In the second dimension, reminders range from optional through "soft-stopped" (requiring at least a simple override) to "hard-stopped"(requiring a specific type of action before anything else can be done).

We know very little about which type of reminder is most effective for what sort of clinical situation. This is partly because so many factors influence reminder effective-

TABLE 9.1. Examples of CDS Reminder Types.

	Intrusive	Non-intrusive
Optional	n/a	Links to clinical guidelines
Soft stopped	A reminder of a potential drug-drug interaction obscures the screen, but can be overridden with a single mouse click.	A button changes color, indicating that preventive care is due soon. An intrusive, soft-stopped reminder fires if the after-visit summary is printed before the reminder is acted on.
Hard-stopped	A reminder that a medicine cannot be ordered without an associated diagnosis obscures the screen until an acceptable diagnosis is entered.	A field turns yellow, indicating that a drug order needs refill information. An intrusive, hard-stopped reminder fires if the user tries to sign the orders before filling in the field.

ness. For an intrusive reminder to be effective, it will need to fire at the right moment. This moment will be after the physician has had a chance to review the information needed to respond to the reminder—unless the reminder contains within itself all the information that will be needed. On the other hand, the reminder will need to be triggered before ordering is complete. Similarly, a non-intrusive reminder can range from hard-to-see (a few small letters turning from black to red) to highly visible (a one-inch button flashing optic yellow and Internet blue). (See Chapter 7.) Linking reminders to order sets with the recommended interventions defaulted is likely to make both types more effective. Reminders that reflect local physician consensus, that are clearly stated, that do not require a change in practice, and that are evidence-based are also more likely to be accepted (4).

Beyond the characteristics of the reminder itself, the presence or absence of effective performance audits and financial incentives largely determines whether reminders are seen as an aid to improved performance or new, unreimbursed work to be avoided.

CDS Performance Standards

We believe that optimal reminders are

- Non-intrusive and highly visible
- Soft stopped
- Fast
- Simple
- Presented just in time
- Actionable (with order sets included in them or linked to them)
- Supported by best evidence, local consensus, payer incentives, and rapid-cycle feedback to individual physicians and their leaders

If you are choosing an EHR, assess carefully how it will enable you to meet these standards.

Fast

Physicians are time pressured. Genuinely effective tools make doing the right thing easier and faster. Order sets and single orders with the (usually) appropriate selection defaulted are particularly effective. So are note templates with the most frequently appropriate response defaulted. CDS messages should be short and clear. Overhage, et al., recommend against complete sentences and correct grammar in favor of messages such as "treat with ACE inhibitor because of diabetes and HTN" (5)—but note that "Consider ACE inhibitor for diabetes and HTN." may actually read faster because the capital "C" and the period cue the eye to the beginning and end of the message.

Simple

Very few providers will use complex tools, whether order sets or note templates. This is true even of well-made tools (5, 6). It is true even of tools they create themselves.

Just in Time

Intrusive reminders, particularly, must be delivered precisely when they are needed. If a reminder can only be presented at the beginning of a patient visit, the provider—having not yet reviewed the problem list and medication list—will not be prepared to respond. Over time, many providers train themselves to ignore such alerts. If the reminder can only be presented after the physician has decided on a course of action and recommended it to the patient, it is likely to be ignored (See Box).

Way Too Late

For approximately one year, we provided intrusive, soft-stopped reminders of primary-care tests and treatments that should precede referrals (for example, osteoarthritis of the knee). Physicians found the content of the reminders clinically appropriate but disliked the reminders so much that we removed them from the EHR. This was because the only available trigger for firing the reminder was ordering the referral. Since the physician has often discussed the referral with the patient before entering the order, following the reminder's advice means that the physician would have to explain that the computer had just informed her that a referral was not yet appropriate because potentially useful primary-care tests and/or treatments should be tried first. Understandably, physicians found being "corrected by the computer" in this very visible way intolerable.

Actionable

In the case of diabetes and HTN, the reminder should include a form for ordering the ACE inhibitor that best fits the patient's formulary—in the dose appropriate to the patient's renal function. (As a first step, there should be a link to an order form pre-filled with the starting dose of the ACE inhibitor that is most frequently prescribed in the practice.)

Managing CDS

In most CDOs, CDS topics have been developed *ad hoc*, driven by the early requirements of payers and regulators and the concerns of local stakeholders. Even in the most advanced organizations, such as the Regenstrief Institute and Kaiser, scheduled review of existing CDS rules is the exception (7). The need to implement and maintain increasing numbers of CDS rules to meet quality and efficiency goals means that all CDOs will need a more organized approach to planning, developing, and maintaining their CDS tools. The Decision Support Implementers' Workbook (8) is a succinct, practical, and thorough guide to this process. It offers step-by-step guidance and useful tools for identifying CDS stakeholders and goals; selecting CDS interventions; developing, testing and launching the interventions; and monitoring and enhancing their effects. This chapter will not duplicate the Workbook's contents. Instead, we will highlight some specific lessons we have learned.

Multidisciplinary Oversight Team

Even a high-performance EHR will have many idiosyncrasies that complicate the development of CDS. For instance, an intrusive reminder might be able to include an order set within it, while a non-intrusive reminder might not support even a link to an order set. Including members of the EHR technical team (who understand these idiosyncrasies) on the CDS oversight team improves the team's efficiency at selecting CDS interventions that are both clinically valuable and technically feasible. The other members of the team will develop considerable expertise at feasibility assessment over time, but normal turnover and the continuing evolution of the EHR's capabilities make ongoing technical team participation necessary.

Clinical Domain Experts

As the outpatient implementation progressed, we came to recognize a constellation of factors that regularly limit the effectiveness of CDS efforts:

- Lack of user awareness of CDS tools (such as note templates and order sets)
- Tools that fit the workflows of one or a few users rather than supporting practice-wide (or organization-wide) needs
- Tools that were built before we learned to make them optimally efficient and flexible
- Tools too large and complex for even the author to use

We concluded that the most efficient way to create and maintain the scores of EHR tools that each practice needs for optimal performance was to enlist a clinical Domain Expert (DE) to lead each practice's CDS tool building. We invite each practice's clinical leader to name a DE for the practice, based on the criteria in the box. We ask the leader to enable the DE to attend an all-day workshop six times a year and to support the DE's work by making activities 1, 2, 3, and 5 a regular part of practice meetings and work expectations for the practice. (Although they are not paid for this work, DEs, most of whom are physicians, receive 6 hours of CME credit for each workshop.)

Anything But a Geek

The ideal Domain Expert possesses the following attitudes, abilities, and skills:

- A deep and broad understanding of the thought processes, common language, workflows, and information needs of a practice
- The respect of the work group—as a practitioner and group member
- A keen understanding of the need for usability, that is, of the most users' limited interest in EHRs for their own sake
- The ability to enlist the aid of fellow-workers in developing and critiquing EHR tools
- The ability to motivate fellow workers to use the EHR effectively
- An understanding of the difference between what is possible with EHRs and what is feasible in the present project—and a willingness to work on achieving the feasible

Clinical-Domain Expert Responsibilities

1. **Identify the practice workflow** most in need of standardization and automation (working with all stakeholders).
2. **Define a standardized workflow**, including information content (working with all stakeholders and explicitly including the best available evidence).
3. *Identify goals and objectives, measures, and the report format for assessing the new process and EMR tools (calling on the informatician mentor for support as needed).*
4. **Build EHR tools** to support the standardized workflow (calling on the informatician mentor for support as needed).
5. **Facilitate stakeholder review** of proposed tools (working with the practice leader)
6. *Report on the effects of the new EHR tools to practice leaders and to the Chief Medical Information Officer (CMIO).*
7. **Identify the next clinical workflow** most in need of standardization and automation.

(Without completion of tasks 3 and 6, the practice will not learn valuable lessons about the effect of their EMR-related improvement efforts, creating the risk of substantial resource waste. On the other hand, resource constraints may make completion of tasks 3 and 6 difficult. For these reasons, measurement and reporting should be as focused and automated as possible, e.g., automated reports on how many times each tool is used will be provided by the EHR technical team.)

EHR Team Support

The EHR team provides the following services to DEs:

1. Introductory and ongoing tool-building education for Clinical-Domain Experts (at bimonthly workshops).

2. An informatician mentor to be consulted as needed.
3. Technical support for tool implementation in the EHR.

Results

We have more than 30 DEs, with 20 to 25 attending each workshop. Each workshop runs from 9 A.M. to 4 P.M.—although many DEs work considerably later—and consists of four 15-minute teaching sessions punctuating long periods for tool building. By the second workshop, the DEs are teaching each other novel solutions to tool building needs, so much so that we have made the sharing of these solutions a standard part of the teaching sessions. Individual DEs routinely build six or more tools during a single workshop. We are not yet able to monitor the use of the tools, but practices report finding the DE's tools very useful.

Our next challenge is to integrate the work of DEs more effectively with practice performance-improvement initiatives. This will require many practices to adopt more formal quality-improvement methodologies as a first step.

Standardization and Freedom

Many organizations (including ours) encourage physicians to develop their own note templates and order sets as a way of increasing physician acceptance of the EHR. We are not aware of even anecdotal evidence that this freedom is important to any but a handful of physicians. The pervasiveness of this strategy is probably due to the fact that clinician members of implementation teams and feedback groups tend to have a strong personal interest in developing software tools. At some point in the implementation, our clinical and administrative leaders and the implementation team become aware that, without standardization, the EHR's support of improved efficiency and quality will be hobbled. For example, if users can edit an evidence-based admission order set, DVT prophylaxis might disappear. In addition, clinicians will lose the efficiencies that come with being able to anticipate standard patterns of care, for example, for uncomplicated open-heart surgery. Finally, the chance of error increases as process variability increases (9).

Identifying three categories of CDS content makes the balancing of standardization and freedom more manageable:

- Organizational standards: These standards represent the organization's understanding of evidence-based best practices, combined with external standards (legal, regulatory, and reimbursement). If one of these standards is not met, the reason must be documented.
- Organizational Conventions: These are conventions the organization has created for the sake of consistency and efficiency. Documenting reasons for non-adherence aids in reviewing and refining the conventions.
- Departmental Conventions: These are similar to organizational conventions, but are relevant only to the work of a single work group.

Flexible Standardization

Healthcare's understanding of process standardization is powerfully conditioned by its continuing dependence on paper records. Since it is rarely feasible to create paper note templates or order sets that support both standardization and flexibility in usably compact form, we are prone to assume that we must choose between standardization and flexibility.

One of the yet-to-be implemented potentials of the EHR is to inform users clearly which elements of a note template or order set represent organizational performance standards (e.g., by highlighting them in yellow) and which are acceptable options. The EHR can also enable the user to document the contraindication to standards they do not perform and the indication for options selected. This ability means that 100% performance, defined as guidance implemented + guidance contraindication documented + patient deferral documented, will become the achievable goal for validated quality measures.

Finally, because patients really are unique, free-text entry should be available in every section of every tool, allowing physicians to adapt their documentation and treatment to the patient's unique needs.

Error as a Source for CDS

Participation of the CDS team in your organization's error-reduction efforts can produce several benefits. One is to sensitize the CDS team to the different types and sources of errors that your organization is addressing. Harnessing the EHR to help prevent these errors (as in the Cortisporin example in Chapter 7 and the methotrexate example below) will provide some of the short-term wins that help to maintain the organization's commitment to the EHR and to CDS. Informatician participation in formal root-cause analyses of errors is particularly productive. (See Glossary.)

Implicit CDS

The EHR provides many opportunities to provide decision support in ways that are minimally intrusive. For example, simply defaulting the new preferred administration rate of a medicine can change prescribing patterns rapidly and dramatically. (6) Changing the order-entry name of a medication (e.g. from "CORTISPORIN OT" to "CORTISPORIN OTIC SUSP (FOR PERFORATION)" can help even specialists prescribe more appropriately (see Chapter 7). Creating pre-populated administration fields for a drug like methotrexate (e.g. "Methotrexate 2.5 mg; four pills together each week") can help avoid prescriptions such as "Methotrexate 2.5 mg; as directed"—and the tragedies that can result from the resulting patient confusion (10). Inserting generic drugs into listings of brand name drugs can aid providers who want to order generic drugs but have trouble remembering their names. For example, if a provider types "lasix", the following list appears:

Lasix (Furosemide 20 mg)
Lasix (Furosemide 40 mg)
Lasix (Furosemide 80 mg)
Lasix 20 mg
Lasix 40 mg
Lasix 80 mg

Transparency and Feedback

It is important to publish in advance (to all users who will be affected), every signifi-cant new CDS intervention. This can be done via E-mail with a link to a Web page. Despite our initial concerns about opening the oversight team to personal attacks, this process produces feedback that has saved us from several implementation errors and increased physician acceptance of CDS. (As physician acceptance of CDS grows, this publication needs to become increasingly selective to avoid irritating physicians with what they have come to regard as routine information.)

Summary

Providing high-quality clinical decision support is difficult but has enormous potential to improve healthcare efficiency and quality. It begins with an EHR designed to support it. It requires agreement regarding CDS opportunities. It demands a steady focus on simple, usable tools that meet the felt needs of physicians and that can be built in the current version of the EHR. It needs ongoing feedback from users regarding what actu-ally supports and what subverts their clinical decision-making.

References

1. Bates DW, Gawande AA. Improving safety with information technology. *New Engl J Med* 2003;348:2526–2534.
2. McGlynn EA, Asch SM, Adams J. The quality of health care delivered to adults in the United States. *New Engl J Med* 2003;348:2635–2645.
3. Yarnall K, Pollak K, Ostbye T. Primary care: is there enough time for prevention? *Am J Public Health* 2003;93(4):635–641.
4. Grol R. Attributes of clinical guidelines that influence use of guidelines in general practice: observational study. *Br Med J* 1998;317:858–861.
5. Overhage J, Tierney W, McDonald C. Clinical decision support: tools, trials, and tribulations. *J Healthcare Inform Manag* 1999;13(2):67.
6. Bates DW, Kuperman GJ, Wang S, Middleton B. Ten commandments for effective clinical decision support: making the practice of evidence-based medicine a reality. *JAMIA* 2003; 10:523–530.
7. Overhage J, Sittig D. CDS rules management. Personal communication; 2003.
8. Content Matrix in the The Decision Support Implementers' Workbook. In: www.himss.org/asp/cds_workbook.asp.
9. Reason J. *Human Error*. Cambridge: Cambridge Univ Press; 1990.
10. Mayor S. UK introduces measures to reduce errors with methotrexate. *Br Med J* 2003;327:70.

Additional Reading

Osheroff J, Sittig D., et al. (2003). Decision-Support Implementer's Workbook. www.himss.org/ASP/cds_workbook.asp
A succinct, practical, thorough guide to getting CDS into practice.
Reason J. (1990). *Human Error*. Cambridge: Cambridge University Press.
The seminal work on the types and causes of error. Must reading for understanding error prevention.

10
Translating Scope of Practice into Effective EHR Workflows

Janet S. Byron, Edward J. Zych, Tracey W. Wolf, and W. Todd Gibson

This chapter provides a methodology for developing EHR access profiles (that is, the level of EHR access, ability to enter information, ability to order tests and treatments, required co-signs, and audit functions) that will assure that all EHR users (including trainees and students), have appropriate access to the EHR, in compliance with regulatory and licensing requirements, (i.e., scope of practice), while maximizing operational efficiency.

A Caveat

The EHR software that Geisinger uses—EpicCare®—provides a specific set of options for integrating the work of the healthcare team. In addition, the regulations that govern supervisory workflows vary from jurisdiction to jurisdiction. In this chapter, we have tried to address healthcare team integration in a general way that will be useful to you, regardless of your location and the software you use. You will, of course, want to carefully review your options, using the elements of our methodology that seem useful for creating a system adapted to your situation.

Background

American healthcare is currently delivered by an increasingly diversified team of caregivers. The effective scope of practice for these caregivers is defined by complex regulations, payer requirements and the policies (explicit and implicit) of individual organizations. The definitions of scope of practice for different caregiver types were created independently and frequently conflict. Over time, clinicians and CDOs have created their own local understandings. That these various understandings are at all workable is due in large part to the ability of "fuzzy" human logic to reconcile conflicting demands. In contrast, the computer requires unambiguous instructions. In the EHR, the ability to view information, enter information, order tests and treatments, and prescribe medications must be precisely defined for each type of clinician.

One of the critical challenges and opportunities of implementing an EHR is the task of defining the scope of practice and the supervisory relationships of each distinct type of caregiver in the organization and then translating these definitions into your EHR system build.

Setting the Stage

Geisinger's EHR implementation began in our freestanding primary-care practices. Prior to the EHR implementation, each practice had maintained its own set of paper medical records. Since these practices were not supervised by the Geisinger Medical Record Practice Committee (MRPC), the Joint Commission for the Accreditation of Healthcare Organizations (JCAHO), or the Pennsylvania Department of Health (DOH), each practice's clinical and administrative leaders decided supervisory workflows that were appropriate for each type of clinician.

In contrast, the practices located on the Geisinger Medical Center campus are designated as hospital outpatient clinics. As such, they are regulated by our MRPC, JCAHO, and the DOH, as well as the Accreditation Council for Graduate Medical Education (ACGME). Complicating matters further, physicians-in-training, psychologists and other mental health professionals, clinical nurse specialists, and various types of ancillary personnel provide patient care in these clinics. We realized that the supervisory workflows appropriate to many of these clinician types required analysis and in some cases redefinition. Further, we saw that many of our decisions made during primary-care EHR implementations were based on misunderstandings of regulatory and payer requirements. Finally, no single individual or department had sufficient knowledge to create policies and procedures that would be both externally valid and operationally workable.

The Healthcare Team Integration Committee

In response to these needs, a multidisciplinary committee was charged with creating appropriate supervisory workflows for implementation in the EHR. This committee is comprised of representatives of the following work groups: physicians, medical educators, legal services, medical records, professional reimbursement and corporate compliance, nursing, residents, physician assistants, and the EHR team. Representatives of individual practices are often invited to provide in-depth information on their practice operations. An experienced EHR project team leader chairs the committee. The CMIO serves as the committee's executive sponsor.

The team was formed at the beginning of the implementation of specialty outpatient practices and continued to meet every two weeks during implementation. As the outpatient implementation concluded, the team turned its attention to the inpatient implementation.

Decision-Making Considerations

In addition to addressing the needs of multiple stakeholders, the committee's decision making must take into account:

1. Existing organizational policies
2. Deeply ingrained work practices that may not be consistent with the policies of the organization—or even of individual practices
3. Increasing financial pressures that make the introduction of workflow inefficiencies unacceptable

Some of the committee's decisions have been dictated unambiguously by regulatory requirements. Most, however, require balancing patient safety, care quality, workflow efficiency, and billing needs. The complexity of these decisions makes sustained involvement of organizational stakeholders and frequent communication with individual practices critical to the committee's success.

Reporting

It is not feasible for the committee to report all of its decisions to oversight forums. The committee is empowered to create and implement policies without further confirmation, particularly where the decision is clear-cut—that is, decisions dictated by a regulation of the DOH, JCAHO, Medicare, or the ACGME. The committee consults one or more of its oversight forums when a decision cannot be made on the basis of a clear regulation and has the potential either to create workflow inefficiencies or is needed to reduce the organization's legal or financial risk. The committee's executive sponsor, the CMIO, helps with these assessments. The CMIO informs the committee's oversight forums (Clinical Operations, Administrative Operations) of the issues the committee has identified and the policy decisions that are needed to guide and support the committee's work. This two-way communication secures the leadership support that is often critical to ensure that new policies and procedures are enacted.

The committee refers an issue to one or more of the oversight forums for advice or final decision about once a month. The committee provides a concise description of the issue, available options, a recommended course of action, and justifications supporting the recommendation. The oversight forums then make the decision, communicate it, and put it into practice.

Documentation

Because of the number, complexity, and sensitivity of decisions made by the committee, thorough written documentation of the decisions, and the reasons for making them, is particularly important. The committee and others refer to this documentation frequently.

Practice Settings

The committee identified three distinct practice settings:

- Freestanding physician practices
- Hospital outpatient clinics
- Hospital inpatient units

The committee postponed all inpatient decisions until the inpatient implementation, although it did consider the inpatient implications of decisions related to outpatient care. Although freestanding and hospital-based outpatient clinics were not (at the time of the committee's work) governed by the same regulatory and payer rules, the committee looked for opportunities to adopt unified policies whenever possible.

EHR Access

Defining user access to various functions of the EHR—through security class assignments in the system build—is a key component of the committee's work. Every potential EHR user type (clinical and non-clinical) needs to have its rights and responsibilities spelled out.

Medication Orders

We define a medication-authorizing provider as an EHR user with authority to give final authorization for a medication order. In the case of paper prescriptions, the medication-authorizing provider's name prints on the prescription for signature by that provider.

Our EHR software divides medication ordering into three parts: (1) initiation, (2) release for action, and (3) final authorization. The following algorithm helps the committee determine the appropriate level of functionality to assign to each caregiver type.

1. Does this caregiver type have a business need and the authority to order medications?
   a. If **NO**, the user can only view the Medications List.
   b. If **YES,**
2. Can this caregiver type initiate orders and release them?
   a. If **NO**, the user will only be able to prepare the medication order for another provider to approve.
   b. If **YES,**
3. Can this caregiver type initiate and release orders and provide final authorization?
   a. If **NO**, the order is automatically routed to the person identified in the EHR as the medication-authorizing provider for her co-signature. The order is released prior to final authorization.
   b. If **YES,**
4. Can this caregiver type provide final authorization for controlled substances?
   a. If **NO**, the order is automatically routed to the medication-authorizing provider for co-sign.
   b. If **YES,**
5. A co-signer is not required.

Exceptions to Every Rule

We found two situations to which this algorithm does not apply. In Pennsylvania, physician assistants (PAs) practicing under the supervision of a physician with an MD license and Clinical Registered Nurse Practitioners (CRNPs) who have been granted prescriptive authority can prescribe medications without a co-signature. However, regulations require that paper prescriptions include the name of the supervising physician.

For this to occur, the security classification of PAs and CRNPs had to be set to require a co-signature on medication orders.

Test Ordering

We define a test-authorizing provider as any caregiver type with the authority to provide final authorization for a diagnostic test. The name of the test-authorizing provider prints on the requisition form with a statement indicating that the order has been electronically authorized.

The following algorithm helps the committee determine the appropriate level of EHR access to assign to each caregiver type:

1. Does this caregiver type have a business need and the authority to order tests?
   a. If **NO**, the user can prepare the test orders for another provider to approve and finalize. If **YES**,
2. Can this caregiver type initiate orders, release orders, and provide final authorization?
   a. If **NO**, the order is automatically routed to a test-authorizing provider for co-signature. Order release is not delayed while the order awaits final authorization.
   b. If **YES**, this caregiver can provide final authorization for test orders; a co-signature is not required.

More Exceptions

Some caregiver types need to place orders exclusively for the purpose of documenting patient services that they have performed. For example, a registered dietitian may be required by payers to enter an order for nutritional services in order to bill for those services. We concluded (with executive concurrence) that requiring a co-signature for these orders would add no quality to care and have no patient safety value. Since our EHR software does not let us limit authorization of orders to a subset of orders, these user types were granted comprehensive ordering ability without the requirement of a co-signature. The leaders of departments affected by these decisions agree in writing to ensure that their staff will order only this limited set of billing codes. To assure compliance, an audit report is forwarded to our internal audit department monthly.

Order Modification

Paper orders can be fairly generic (e.g., "ultrasound to rule out kidney stones") and the physician performing the procedure (or their support staff) has considerable latitude in translating the order into the procedure (and code) that is ultimately performed and billed. For example, an order for a cardiac stress test may use either exercise or a pharmacologic stressor and either ultrasound or radioisotope photography. The need for modification is particularly true with radiology tests, where the optimal test for answering a specific diagnostic question (and its availability) may change frequently.

The decision of the physician performing the test to discuss such modifications with the ordering physician is based on a complex and largely implicit set of criteria, including the radiologist's working relationship with the ordering provider. Many radiology orders are treated as consults—as if the order read, "Use the most appropriate test to assess whether this patient has kidney stones."

The EHR's requirement of precise instructions raised several questions:

1. On what basis may the original order be modified?
2. Does the ordering provider need to approve the modification before the test is performed?
3. Does the ordering provider want to be consulted if the order is modified?
4. Who is responsible for the test that is finally performed—the physician who gave the original order, or the performing provider who modified the original order?

To answer this set of questions:

1. We created some orders that are flexible by definition. One is the above example of cardiac stress testing. A provider may order a specific test (e.g., pharmacologic stress echo) or order a generic cardiac stress test, leaving it to the physician who performs the test to decide which form of stress and which type of photography are most appropriate.

2. Practice managers and the EHR training curricula encourage ordering providers to use the "Order Detail" field to specify their clinical question and to indicate if modifications of the order are acceptable.

3. Radiology leadership reinforces the need for test-performing physicians to check with the ordering physician if a proposed order modification is substantial. (According to Medicare regulations, a radiologist is permitted to change a physician's order without first contacting the ordering physician when changing a non-contrast study to a contrast study (and vice versa) and when changing a screening mammogram to a diagnostic mammogram.)

Supervision Requirements

Aside from determining ordering capabilities for caregiver types, you will also need to decide who can practice independently and who requires supervision. Supervision is mandated by the ACGME for resident physicians and fellows. With respect to supervision requirements, the ACGME considers fellows as equivalent to residents. (Fellows are included with residents throughout this discussion.) Medicare billing requirements may necessitate additional supervision.

The committee asked five questions to characterize each caregiver type's need for supervision:

1. Which caregiver types may provide supervision?
2. Which caregiver types require supervision?
3. What type of supervision must each caregiver type receive?
4. Which (if any) work types need to be sent automatically to a supervising provider for review?
   a. Test results?
   b. Patient encounter documentation?
5. Do the caregiver types' transcribed documents require review and counter-signature by a supervising physician?

In answer to the first question, the committee concluded that in Pennsylvania, only a physician (MD or DO) may serve as a supervising provider, with the single exception that a PhD psychologist may supervise psychiatric clinical social workers and psychiatric clinical nurse specialists.

In response to the second and third questions, the committee established three types of supervision: direct, general and moonlighting resident. (Note that the definitions of direct and general supervision are different for residents and mid-level providers.)

A. Supervision of Residents

Direct: The supervising physician must personally see and examine the patient. The medical record documentation must attest to this fact.

General: The supervising physician discusses the case with the resident or lets the resident act independently, but is available for consultation.

B. Supervision of Mid-level Providers

Direct: The supervising physician (with whom the mid-level has a written collaborative agreement) must be physically located within the practice area and be available to offer immediate assistance.

General: The supervising physician must be available to discuss the care of the patient (e.g., via phone or two-way radio). The mid-level's documentation must refer to any conversation with the supervising physician.

C. Supervising Moonlighting Residents

Under specific circumstances, a resident can practice independently in an outpatient clinic during hours that are outside of the scope of the residency program. When serving in this capacity, the resident is no longer bound by the supervision requirements of the residency program.

Managing Preliminary Reports

Because of the time-sensitive nature of many clinical documents, when a document is sent to the EHR via the transcription interface, it becomes available for review immediately. At this point, the document is prominently labeled as "***DRAFT REPORT***." It also contains the message, "***DICTATED, NOT ELECTRONICALLY SIGNED***," reinforcing the warning that it still requires review and electronic signature.

When an author whose documentation requires a co-signature signs the document, the "DRAFT" label is replaced with the following text—"***Pending Supervising Physician's Review***." This phrase is visible on the "Results Review" screen, which provides the initial access point for most users. After he authenticates the document, the author forwards the document to the supervising physician's in-basket. After the supervising physician authenticates (co-signs) the document (with or without electronic edits), it is final and is displayed without any qualifying label.

Delegated Order Entry

In many of our practices, process efficiency has long been dependent on support staff ordering diagnostic tests (under both explicit and implicit protocols). This practical business need conflicts directly with a primary goal of EHR implementation, which is to assure that all of the alerts and reminders triggered by an order are considered by the ordering provider prior to the order's release.

We did not want to degrade efficiency in practices where diagnostic studies routinely need to be done before the physician sees the patient (e.g., a patient in orthopedics clinic with a suspected ankle fracture). Based on our review of billing requirements and Pennsylvania regulations, some tests may be ordered by nurses—if they are ordered under a written protocol, under a physician's supervision, and with a physician's timely co-signature.

Since practices already had follow-up order sets for all of their commonly seen problems (e.g., ankle fracture follow-up), an EHR exception was needed only for patients with new problems. Some practices (e.g., orthopedics and nephrology) have developed practice-specific protocols under which nurses order specific tests for patients with new problems. The physician co-signs the order at the same time that she documents the visit and orders follow-up testing.

Prescription Renewals

The Pennsylvania State Board of Medicine considers the renewal of a medication to be a new act of prescribing, regardless of how long a patient has been taking the medication. A telephoned prescription or renewal is legal only if it is based on the input and judgment of an individual "properly authorized to issue a prescription". This means that practice staff—unlicensed or licensed—cannot call in a new prescription or a renewal without prior authorization from an individual with prescriptive authority. To communicate this throughout the organization, the Department of Legal Services developed and published a prescription renewal policy.

Prescription Renewal Policy

In a clinic or physician office, a telephone call to a pharmacy for the placement of a new prescription medication order or the renewal of a chronic prescription medication can be placed by office support staff, *if and only if*, there has been prior verbal or written authorization for the placement of this medication order by an individual who has been granted prescriptive authority.

The State Board of Medicine will not condone the delegation of prescriptive authority to the office support staff through the use of protocols that are developed for the purpose of allowing office staff to order or renew medications without first obtaining authorization from someone with prescriptive authority.

This restriction shall not apply to a nationally recognized treatment protocol or one that is in widespread use for reasons other than the convenience of the prescribing provider. Failure to comply with these requirements is considered the unauthorized practice of medicine and will be prosecuted as such by the State Board of Medicine.

In the standard workflow, practice support staff (clerical or nursing) document the patient's request for the prescription renewal and initiate the order in the EHR. They then route the request to a provider who has prescriptive authority. The provider authorizes the order and routes the encounter back to the support staff. If there is an urgent need for a medication, support personnel need verbal authorization for the renewal. Verbal authorization is documented in the EHR using the standard phrase:

"A verbal authorization to renew the medication(s) was obtained, as well as permission to communicate the authorization directly to the pharmacy."

Out-of-Office Coverage

When a provider is going to be unavailable for patient care, it is standard practice to designate a covering provider. Our EHR software allows for test results and patient calls that arrive during a provider's absence to be routed automatically to another provider's in-basket. The provider who will be out designates a covering provider in the EHR and sets the effective dates. The out of office provider also determines whether:

1. Results and messaging should be routed to the covering provider's inbasket exclusively, or
2. Results and messages should be routed to the covering provider's inbasket and to the out of office provider's inbasket.

Providers must sign out to providers with equivalent licensure and scope of practice or to a physician (Table 10.1).

In extraordinary circumstances, a physician may sign out to a PA or a CRNP. In these cases, the physician is required to receive a copy of all test results, patient calls and medication requests in his inbasket.

To Pool or Not to Pool?

Initially, our EHR software only allowed a provider to select another individual provider to serve as the covering provider. Later, a software upgrade enabled routing of information to caregiver pools. Pools have the advantage of allowing several workers to share the management of the information. For example, a message sent to a nursing pool or clerical pool can be managed by whichever pool member is available. This arrangement decreases the likelihood that a message will languish in the inbasket of an absent caregiver, decreases the turnaround time for patient requests, and allows for workload smoothing. There are, however, significant risks associated with pools. Given that our EHR system does not restrict who can be in a pool, it would be possible for the provider to select a provider pool that did not include any members. Additionally, even if the pool included providers, it would still be possible for a result to be reviewed and deleted by a user who was not a provider. (When a message is deleted from a pool, the information is removed from the inbasket of every user participating in the pool.)

For these reasons and because of our organization's requirement that results be reviewed and signed by a physician, the committee concluded that, "A provider shall not designate pools of EHR users to be responsible for reviewing test results and patient requests in the provider's absence."

TABLE 10.1. Providers with Equivalent Licensure and Scope of Practice:

- Physician to physician
- Fellow to fellow
- PA to PA
- CRNP to CRNP
- Resident Year 1 to any level resident
- Residents Year 2–5 to Residents Year 2–5
- Pharmacist to Pharmacist (only)
- PhD Psychologist to PhD Psychologist
- Nurse Midwife to Nurse Midwife

Mid-level Providers

We have identified these types of mid-level providers in our organization: Physician Assistant (PA), Certified Registered Nurse Practitioner (CRNP), Clinical Nurse Specialist, Clinical Social Worker, Psychologist, Optometrist, Certified Nurse Anesthetist, and Certified Nurse Midwife. The scope of practice of mid-level providers is complex. For example, CRNPs are regulated by the Pennsylvania Boards of Nursing, Medicine, and Pharmacy, as well as the Department of Health.

Psychologists cannot write orders for medications and are not allowed to order tests or procedures. On the other hand, psychologists function independently with regard to the therapy they provide to patients. This means that their EHR access in some areas will be similar to that of physicians, while in other areas they will have limited access. These distinctions create considerable irritation among some EHR users. Clinical nurse specialists and psychologists often work as partners with physicians and expect their EHR access to reflect this. Unfortunately, laws and regulations may make supervision by a physician mandatory. Since reviewing test results and cosigning the orders and clinical notes of mid-levels may represent new work for supervising physicians, the physicians may also resist the changes. This is one of the places where multidisciplinary input and strong executive support are especially important.

When Pennsylvania-based mid-level providers order tests and procedures, they work under a different set of regulations in an outpatient practice not associated with a hospital than in a practice associated with a hospital. This affects requirements for supervision and billing. Because mid-levels' scope of practice is dependent on the practice setting, we analyzed functionality needs at the individual practice level. Central questions were:

1. What (if any) medications may they order? With or without co-signature?
2. What test and procedures may they order? With or without co-signature?
3. Do their clinical observations require a co-signature?
4. Can they supervise other caregiver types?

The committee's decisions are reflected in the Mid-Level EHR Functionality Table (see Table 10.2).

Residents and Fellows

The ACGME and the JCAHO define appropriate supervision of graduate medical trainees, such as residents and fellows. Central questions are:

TABLE 10.2. Mid-Level Provider EHR Functionality Table.

Provider Type	Medication Authorizing Provider?	Orders Authorizing Provider?	Can you serve as a Supervising Provider?	Do You Require Supervision?	Do you require a co-sign for dictated documents?	Auto CC of the Chart?	Auto CC of the Results?
Physician Assistant	**Yes** From a Security Class perspective, we have to require a co-sign in order to have the name of the co-signing physician also print on their script form.	**Yes without Co-sign**	No	Yes	Yes	Yes	Yes
PhD Psychologist	No	**Yes without Co-sign**	Yes	Optional	No	N/A	N/A
Certified Registered Nurse Practitioner (CRNP)	**Setting this to be Yes or No** depends upon the Prescriptive Authority per the CRNP's Collaborative Practice Agreement. From a Security Class perspective, we have to require a co-sign in order to have the name of the co-signing physician also print on their script form.	**Yes without Co-sign**	No	**Yes** This is a billing requirement.	**No** Clin Ops Decision 1/22/02	**No** Clin Ops Decision 1/22/02	**No** Clin Ops Decision 1/22/02
Clinical Nurse Specialist (CNS)	No	**Yes with Co-sign**	No	Yes	No	**No** Clin Ops Decision 3/05/02	**Yes**
Certified Nurse Midwife (CNM)	No	**Yes without Co-sign**	No	**Yes** This is a billing requirement	**No** The CNMs are only dictating correspondence, not patient care documentation.	No	No
Optometrists	**If the 't' suffix is present in the Optometrist's license number, then set to YES for Meds Authorizing, otherwise set to NO.**	**Yes without Co-sign**	No	No	N/A	N/A	N/A

1. What are the supervision requirements for physicians-in-training with unrestricted licenses?
2. What are the implications of DEA certification and its absence?
3. Can residents or fellows supervise other caregiver types?
4. How does "moonlighting" status affect supervision requirements?

Our answers are as follows:

1. All residents and fellows must have their patients' test results and documentation reviewed by a supervising physician. Their orders do not require a co-sign, except as in 2, below.

2. If a physician-in-training does not have a DEA number, he must enter the supervising physician as the physician authorizing for any controlled substance. The supervising provider must sign the electronic prescription and any paper prescription.

3. Residents and fellows provide education and working supervision for junior residents and medical students. This informal supervision must be distinguished from formal supervision, which is the sole responsibility of attending or staff physicians. Neither residents nor fellows can provide formal supervision for other caregiver types or any student.

4. When a resident selects "moonlighting" as her type of supervision (while completing orders or documentation) the requirement for automatic forwarding of the chart and test results is inactivated in the EHR.

Students

For medical, nursing, mid-level (PA and CRNP), pharmacy, audiology, and other allied healthcare students, the questions are these:

1. How will we educate students regarding the importance of preserving patient confidentiality?
2. Can they access test results?
3. Can they order medications? Is a co-signature required?
4. Can they order tests? Is a co-signature required?
5. Can they record clinical observations in the EHR?

Initially, the committee concluded that, since the rotations of medical students, PA students and CRNP students are too short for extensive EHR training, they would be limited to read-only Results Review access. Later, at the request of rotation directors, the committee allowed students to document clinical observations and initiate orders (for a provider to authorize and release). A new security class that includes the ability to initiate (but not release) orders and the ability to record observations in a screen separate from the physician's note meet this need.

Summary

Implementing an EHR will raise scores of questions such as the ones covered in this chapter. Creating a multidisciplinary committee to address them proactively and systematically will increase the efficiency, quality, and financial benefits of your project.

11
System Integration

ELIZABETH A. BOYER, JEAN A. ADAMS, and DIANE L. BARNES

Integrating the EHR, that is, enabling the EHR and other software applications to exchange data with each other without loss of meaning or accuracy, is one of the critical tasks of the EHR implementation and of ongoing production support. Integrating the EHR begins with defining the components to be integrated. The EHR suite is a suite of applications that you purchase from the vendor and that share a common database. It may include scheduling, registration, outpatient EHR, inpatient EHR, Emergency Department EHR, ADT, pharmacy, laboratory billing, and other applications. Ancillary applications are external to the EHR suite, but send information to the suite's database (for example, laboratory and pathology results) and may receive information from it (e.g., patient demographics) (see Figure 11.1).

While part of the value proposition of buying an EHR suite from one vendor is that the suite's components are theoretically integrated from the design stage forward, this is not likely to be entirely the case. So EHR integration has a dual focus: first on establishing interfaces with ancillary applications, and second on integrating data definitions and shared software functions within the EHR suite.

Ancillary Applications

Integration of ancillary applications is essential to the success of the EHR's usability and reliability. Before we implemented the EHR in any practice, we interfaced laboratory results and ancillary patient registration data to the EHR. Radiology results were added early on in the implementation. The advantages of including these data in the EHR include are detailed in Chapter 14.

Considerable back-end work is necessary to make interfaced results from ancillary applications usable:

- Textual reports should display the most pertinent information first (e.g. the impression or final result), with supporting information following. This saves users from having to scroll through at least one screen to view every radiology and pathology result. Since few EHR or ancillary applications were designed with this goal in mind, putting the results first requires extensive manipulation of the incoming data—and is not be feasible in all cases.
- Formatted information displays from ancillary applications should be as readable in the EHR as they are in the originating application. This is often not feasible. In those cases, we import an image of the table into our image-management system and create a link from the EHR to the image.

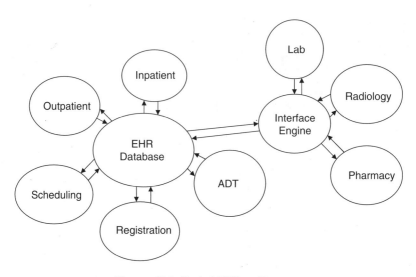

FIGURE 11.1. Typical EHR architecture.

Technical Interface Considerations

- *Decide what data should be stored in the EHR database* and what should remain in ancillary applications. For example, PACS (digital radiology) images are too large to be stored in the EHR. Nor are they needed for real-time transactions (to enable clinical decision support).
- *Document the specifications for each interface.* This documentation should identify each data item and the aggregate data flow. We have learned (from repeated changes in the data needs of various stakeholders) that it is best to interface every data field and then use the interface engine to control which fields actually enter the EHR.
- *Active, continuing management of error logs* is necessary to assure the integrity of the data in the EHR. Our production support team analyzes the logs, designs a process for handling the errors, and designates the team who will monitor the logs and resolve the errors. When the system served only outpatient practices, we monitored the outpatient EHR logs once daily, Monday through Friday. With the implementation of the inpatient EHR, we monitor the logs every four hours, seven days a week.
- *Develop a detailed testing scenario* for every interface message type sent and received. For example,
  - Patient merges, in which the data in duplicate patient records is merged into a single patient record
  - Order and result messages, including different test status indicators (e.g., "In Progress," "Final," "Edited," "Cancelled")
  - Registration messages, including checking a patient in using the scheduling application or making a change to the patient's address

Integrating the EHR Suite

Attention must also be given to data integration among the applications that share the single EHR database (the EHR suite). Detailed analysis needs to confirm that shared data fields have the same definition and use in the various EHR applications before the development, population, and maintenance of data tables. For example, in our EHR the "Department Specialty" field is primarily used and controlled by the scheduling application for managing referrals. Well into the implementation, we discovered that this field is also used as a filter for determining which order sets and note templates various groups of users will see. Had we known this at the outset, we would have placed all our family practitioners in a single Department Specialty. The fact that we created a separate scheduling department for each of the 42 practices requires us to maintain 42 separate lists of order sets and note templates.

Translations may be required from one or more fields in one application to another field in another application. For example, entering the visit type and provider type for an appointment in our scheduling system requires translation to the appropriate encounter type in the EHR (Table 11.1).

Integrated Application Testing

Integrated application testing ensures that new and existing software functions perform well together. The first stage is testing within each application. The second stage is testing the functions across all the applications of the EHR suite. A testing plan will help you identify testing dependencies and prerequisites (see Appendix 7). It will also help you coordinate the necessary resources from the involved project teams (e.g., scheduling and patient care). Table 11.2 provides a guide for estimating testing resource needs.

Scenario-based testing ensures that recommended workflows are functional through-out the EHR suite. For example, does making test ordering easier for generalists make it harder for specialists? Test as many non-recommended workflows as your team can identify to make sure that they do not degrade system performance or cause other kinds of problems. (Of course, users will create far more non-recommended workflows than your testing teams can.)

Master File Management

Populating the EHR's master files (database files that contain static records used to identify, for example, EHR users, work centers, diagnoses or appointment types) appro-priately enables the applications of the EHR suite to work together. We created a

TABLE 11.1. Mapping from Appointment Detail to Encounter Type.

Scheduling Application Convert from	Visit type	Provider type	EHR Encounter type
Appointment	Allergy injection.	Nurse	Nurse only
Appointment	Lab	Nurse	Laboratory
Appointment	Weight check	Nurse	Nurse only
Appointment		Nurse specialist	Office visit
Appointment		Audiologist	Office visit
Appointment		Physician	Office visit

master file team that went through the following steps to populate and maintain the files:

- The vendor identified the files and recommended a methodology for populating them.
- With the vendor's assistance, the team identified the application in the EHR suite (e.g., scheduling, patient-care) that uses the table primarily and controls its definition, along with other applications that use the table.
- The team established and maintained naming conventions that are used throughout the EHR suite. For example, departments are given two-part names, with the specialty followed by the location: "Cardiology—Danville."
- The team determined which master files need to be updated and the methodologies and schedules for those updates. Updates to some master files depend on external application updates. For example, if the laboratory adds, deletes or modifies a test name or number, the procedure and laboratory master files must be changed. Managing updates requires 3 to 4 FTEs. Monthly and annual updates create spikes in demand. See Table 11.3 for a sample schedule of external master file updates.
- The team documents master file changes and communicates them to the implementation, training, and production support teams, who communicate them to the appropriate users. E-mails (with screen shots) are usually adequate, but we present some complex changes in face-to-face demonstrations. The most effective method of recording master file changes for reference is a combination of screen shots and a

TABLE 11.2. Testing Resource Planning Guide.

Type of Project	Resources	Activities	Time Commitment
Development project (e.g. new report)	2 FTEs*	• Double checking of configuration • Testing	Varies based on project complexities.
Monthly updates-annual upgrades	At least 2 FTEs per software application (in our case, 8–10 FTEs for scheduling, registration, ADT, and patient care application.)	• Documentation interpretation • Outline configuration choices for design and feedback groups • System configuration • Test application function • Test application performance • Train users • Implement system • Resolve post-implementation problems	• 6–8 weeks for one monthly update • 12 weeks for 2 monthly updates • 16 weeks for 3 monthly updates
Major upgrade	At least 2 FTEs per application (e.g. 8–10 FTEs)	• Interpret upgrade documentation • Outline configuration choices for design and feedback groups • Configure system • Test application function • Test application performance (simulator) • Train users • Implement system • Resolve post-implementation problems	• 6–12 months based on the size of the upgrade

*2 FTEs are required for any new development project: one primary and one secondary. Two members are needed to provide a comprehensive understanding of the project and for double-checking the configuration settings and testing results.

TABLE 11.3. Schedule of External Master File Updates.

Update Import Type	Frequency	Purpose
Medications	Monthly	Update the EHR with the FDA's most recent approvals. Interaction checking (drug-drug, drug-food, and drug-allergen) is included.
Laboratory	Monthly	Update the EHR with current tests. This includes lab locations and reasons for cancelling tests.
Radiology	Every other month or as needed	Update the EHR with current radiology codes. This allows the radiology results interface to link the result with the order in the EHR.
ICD/CPT/HCPCS	Annually	Update the EHR with current codes.

narrative outlining the options considered, pros and cons identified for each option, reasons for the decision, and stakeholder approval (e.g., feedback groups or leadership teams).

EHR Application Upgrades

Because they affect other EHR applications, large upgrades require a structured approach:

- First, the upgrade team reviews the vendor's upgrade documentation, analyzing functional enhancements and the configuration decisions that will need to be made. They bring any gaps in documentation to the vendor for completion.
- If the upgrade involves more than one application, the upgrade team plans how to integrate configuration and testing of the applications.
- The technical team creates an alternative environment for testing.
- The upgrade team compiles a checklist, which details pre-installation and installation tasks. They complete and document the pre-installation tasks and time the installation steps in order to plan the downtime windows that will be needed for installation.
- The team reviews all of the test environment logs, notes all errors, and presents them to the vendor for resolution. (This is one of the situations where a strong and cooperative partnership with your EHR vendor is most important. You may need them to make changes that you regard as critical before you can implement the upgrade.)
- After the vendor completes the needed improvements, the team installs them in the test environment. Affected application teams are then notified to begin set-up and testing. They apply their upgrade notes, fixes, patches, and enhancements in the test environment and test them thoroughly, with special attention to integrity of data and function across applications.
- Infrastructure components, such as the network, local servers and workstations, are monitored to ensure that the upgrade does not increase network traffic or create software registry incompatibilities. We simulate the number of concurrent users of the production EHR (4100–4500) in the test environment. Specialized testing software simulates standard workflows, tracks the data, and sends it to the vendor for review. If the results indicate that a new or enhanced software function is slowing performance unacceptably, we inactivate it.

- A unified spreadsheet is used to record, prioritize, and monitor the resolution of problems identified by the teams. This spreadsheet is critical for managing the numerous problems that arise, and for communicating with the vendor.
- As testing is completed, the training curriculum is prepared, documentation written, and training classes scheduled.
- As the go-live date approaches, the installation team is informed of the plan and trained in their roles.
- Go-live downtimes are scheduled on weekends (usually Saturday evenings or early Sunday mornings) to minimize the impact on inpatient units, the emergency department, and outpatient practices. During the downtime, the production environment is unavailable to clinical users, but the shadow copy of the EHR (read only and without real-time interfaced results) remains available. As soon as the installation is completed, each application is tested quickly. When the tests are complete, the Help Desk is notified, the interfaces restarted, and user log-ins re-enabled.

On the Monday after go-live, a team of five to ten production support personnel is dedicated full-time to resolving any problems the upgrade has created. Within two to three days, the number of new problems has usually decreased enough to handled by the standard production support processes. All problems are recorded, prioritized, monitored and communicated with the vendor (as appropriate) using the same methodology as for pre-installation testing. Using this methodology, we have shortened the average upgrade installation downtime from eight to three hours.

Summary

Integrating the applications that comprise the EHR application suite and the applications that interface with your EHR is critical to your initial and ongoing success. In many cases, major upgrades can create enough data integrity and usability problems to pose a serious threat to patient safety and workflow efficiency. A thorough, proactive approach to integrating data and functionality across applications will help you minimize this risk.

12
Production Support

ELIZABETH A. BOYER and MICHAEL W. SOBACK

Introduction

At the start of the EHR project, each EHR team member shared in providing production support. Members of the team rotated in a twenty-four hour, seven-days a week on-call schedule. We found that this arrangement compromised productivity by creating both frequent interruptions to project work and post-call fatigue. It also led to employee dissatisfaction, since time spent on production support was not factored into project deadlines and performance goals. As the number of concurrent users increased from hundreds to thousands, these problems became more acute.

To address increased production support needs, we developed a dedicated production support team. This team consists of staff with extensive application and business-process knowledge, as well as customer-relations skills. The primary focus of the team is to handle customer problems. Other tasks include managing user access to the EHR and reviewing daily interface error logs. The errors range from misfiled results—due to ordering errors within the EHR—to invalid interface filing types to patient mismatches and duplicate orders. The team is not responsible for new projects (see Figure 12.1).

The goal of production support is to provide a highly usable, highly available EHR and rapid responses to user problems. Several activities are required to meet this goal: a Help Desk, application-level support, hardware support, and network support. This chapter focuses on efficient organization of these services.

Help Desk

To ensure that requests are handled efficiently and according to the urgency of the need, a priority is assigned to each request at the time the Help Desk receives it. The Help Desk answers questions and fixes problems, when it can. If the Help Desk is unable to fix the problem, they triage the call to the appropriate group. Each call ticket (work-order tracking form) has one of four priority classifications: (1) Routine, (2) Important, (3) Urgent, and (4) Critical. Each priority classification is defined by time-to-resolution performance standards (Table 12.1).

Problem Information Flow

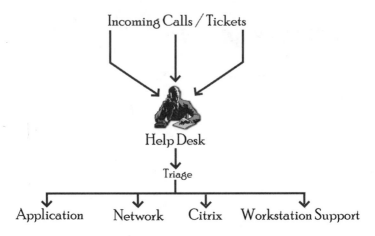

FIGURE 12.1. Production-Support Information Flow.

TABLE 12.1. Problem Status Tracking.

Tracking Status	Description of Status	Customer Requirements	Support goal
Routine	A problem that occurs at random, on occasion, but the device is not completely down	None	1. Respond to ticket within one business day. 2. Resolve ticket within five business days of creation. 3. This priority can be assigned Monday through Friday 8 AM–5 PM.
Important	Indicates a device is completely inoperable, but is not impacting patient care.	None	1. Respond to ticket within four hours. 2. Resolve ticket within one business day of creation. 3. This priority can be assigned Monday through Friday 8 AM–5 PM.
Urgent	Indicates a situation/problem that causes a significant detrimental impact to an individual's or an area's daily responsibility.	1. Requires customer to be on site and available to assist. 2. Customer's manager will be notified if the problem escalates.	1. Respond to ticket within two hours. 2. Resolve ticket within 24 hours of creation. 3. This priority can be assigned 24 × 7 × 365.
Critical	Indicates a problem with a critical device being completely down with no other alternative for a customer where a patient's life is at stake or affects the care given to a patient.	1. Requires customer to be on site and available to assist. 2. Customer's manager will be notified if the problem escalates.	1. Respond to ticket within 30 minutes. 2. Resolve ticket within four hours of creation. 3. This priority can be assigned 24 × 7 × 365.

Skill Sets

Your production support team will need a complex skill set to provide effective help to users. Core skills include triaging calls for network hardware and EHR problems, providing help with Windows applications, and triaging problems related to other applications and interfaces (Table 12.2).

The need for customer-relations skills is a truism. But it is especially necessary for healthcare IT team members. For a variety of reasons, physicians are very sensitive (usually unconsciously) to being in the subordinate position that a student has vis-à-vis a teacher. This means that an IT person helping a physician with a problem may become the brunt of anxieties and anger that the physician is not consciously aware of. This makes the ability to make the customer feel capable a critical skill for these team members.

Geisinger's production support teams provide service to over 40 practice sites in 31 counties. To provide timely support, we have developed a "layered" approach to support, with first-line support (super-users and the Help Desk) available in practice sites, and second-line support (network generalists and workstation and technical analysts) available locally. Third-line support (application support analysts and support consultants) is located centrally. This centralization of back-up support teams enables the frequent face-to-face meetings that are often necessary to solve complex problems.

Communication among all levels of the production support team is critical to effective performance. Frequently updated training for the entire team forms the foundation for communication. In addition, small workgroup meetings, face–to-face meetings with project stakeholders and conference calls are also used to facilitate education and communication (see Figure 12.2).

TABLE 12.2. Skill Set Descriptions.

Skill Set	Role Description	Skills and Behaviors
HelpDesk Staff	The Help Desk staff responds to all IT-related requests for help, phoned and E-mailed. They provide help directly or triage the request to the appropriate team for resolution. Each call is entered as a ticket in an electronic tracking system, which reports time to response and resolution for each ticket.	• Basic application, workstation, and network knowledge • Customer relations skills • Triage appropriately • Know the appropriate teams to receive various help request types • Troubleshoot novel problems • Prioritize and manage multiple requests concurrently
Workstation Analyst	Workstation and technical analysts work in decentralized locations to support individual clinics within the system. They interact directly with the user community.	• Intermediate to advanced workstation hardware skills (personal computers and peripherals) • Intermediate to advanced software/application skills • Proficiency with all utility applications and most other general applications • Troubleshoot problems

TABLE 12.2. *Continued*

Skill Set	Role Description	Skills and Behaviors
Super-user	Super-users are members of clinical teams (e.g., nurses and administrators) who are well trained in the use of the EHR and the specific group's workflows. They provide the first line of production support for their work groups, answering user questions, updating users' training, and serving as liaisons between their work group and the Help Desk. Super-users are trained early in the implementation process. Trainees have access to the EHR in a testing environment so that they can become familiar with optimal EHR workflows.	• A positive, task-oriented approach to problems and to other HER users • Excellent communication skills; friendly and approachable • Teaching skills • Support the quality and efficiency goals of the EHR • Support information security and confidentiality policies • Enable communication between the practice and the EHR support team
Network Generalists	Network generalists are dispersed throughout the system to support clusters of community-based practices. They provide a broad range of IT services, including second-line support for EHR problems. They often work directly with end users.	• Intermediate to advanced workstation hardware skills (personal computers and peripherals) • General network knowledge • Proficiency with all utility applications (e.g., Microsoft Office, GroupWise, Terminal Emulation Package) and most other general applications (e.g., EHR-Epic, Radiology-IDX Rad, Laboratory-Misys) • Conduct regular staff meetings to enlist feedback and communicate updates • Know whom to contact for problems • Basic desktop computer and printer troubleshooting • EHR-related Windows' skills (including keyboard shortcuts) • Basic Internet and billing policies and procedures
Application Support Analysts	These analysts provide the second line of EHR production support behind Super-Users. The group consists of associate, intermediate and senior system analysts who work in a central location. The analysts handle acute as well as routine issues and maintenance tasks. They interact directly with EHR users and all levels of support staff.	• Expert support for selected applications (e.g., EHR outpatient, EHR inpatient, scheduling, registration, ADT) • Basic support for general applications (e.g., Microsoft Office, GroupWise E-mail) • Troubleshoot novel problems • Prioritize and manage multiple tasks concurrently • Research specific problems with the software vendor's support staff
Production Support Consultants	These are lead systems analysts, programmers, and hardware system experts who work in a central location. Their primary focus is the development and implementation of new software applications. They also provide expert consulting support to other production support teams.	• Provide specialized technical expertise • Work effectively with clinicians and administrative leaders • Troubleshoot novel problems • Research specific problems with the software vendor's support staff • Recommend and implement EHR software upgrades • Teach analytical skills to other support team members

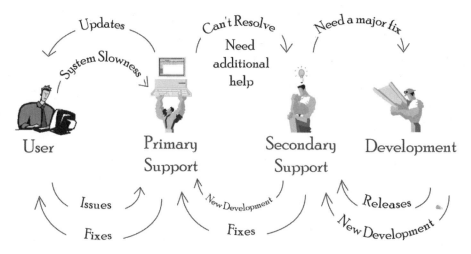

FIGURE 12.2. Production-Support Information Flows.

Unexpected Outcomes

Since separate teams are now responsible for new projects and production support, it is particularly vital for project teams to produce useful written documentation and other forms of communication. They have responded to the challenge with marked improvement. Clear team responsibilities have led to a new sense of purpose and direction on the part of team members. The production support team not only understands the user's need fully, but also is responsible for follow through. This has enabled them to resolve issues more quickly and efficiently.

Skilled listening and problem definition are important in part because many production support calls are, in effect, requests for EHR enhancements, rather than reports of EHR problems. This makes the production support team a valuable source of ideas for project teams.

User Security Set-Up

Initially, two analysts on the EHR team assigned the level of EHR data access (the EHR security set-up) to EHR users. When a user called the Help Desk, the Help Desk staff paged the on-call analyst. The analyst worked with a security administrator to fulfill the request (which could be for anything from resetting a password to troubleshooting a user's inability to access the EHR). As the number of EHR users increased, operational efficiency required that the Help Desk staff and EHR team analysts be able to manage security set-up requests with less direct involvement of security administrators.

To make this possible, the security administrators developed security set-up policies and procedures, credentialing standards, and training materials for the Help Desk staff and the EHR systems analysts who would be providing second-level support (see Appendix 8 for the policies and procedures).

This system has reduced the time it takes to fulfill a request from three hours to 30-minutes. The Help Desk staff are able to fulfill 75% of requests themselves. With this new set of skills the Help Desk has become a cost-effective way to provide rapid support to users during second shift.

Despite its successes, the system did create problems. Errors in user security set-ups caused user dissatisfaction and increased Help Desk calls. We have learned that on-going training and proactive communication among all support groups is critical to maintain consistent performance across this large and varied team. This is particularly true when applications are upgraded or new applications are installed.

Application Upgrade Management

For more information on application upgrade management, see the discussion in Chapter 11.

Summary

Regardless of the details of your organization's production support needs, you will want to pay close attention to many of the themes discussed in this chapter, particularly these:

- Dedicating a team to production support tasks
- Centralizing the team to facilitate knowledge sharing
- Developing strong customer relations skills in the team members
- Rapid, prioritized resolution of user problems
- Cross-training (including the Help Desk) to provide rapid response to common problems
- Specialized teams to provide sophisticated support for complex problems
- Ongoing customer relations training for every team member who works directly with users

13
Managing the Client-Vendor Partnership

FRANK RICHARDS

Introduction

During the 1980s and 1990s, partnerships became a buzzword for a wide variety of business relationships. True business partnerships are built on mutual goals, trust, and the recognition that, for one partner to succeed, both must. Few, if any, information systems acquisitions are as complex or risky to implement as an EHR. Trusting a vendor enough to hand over partial control of your most valuable information assets is not to be taken lightly. Finding the right system with the right capabilities is critical, but finding the right company, one that you can do business with over the long-term, is equally important. This is particularly the case with EHRs, which unlike lab and billing systems are still relatively immature.

Why Is the Client-Vendor Relationship Important?

Most people would agree that you do not need a personal relationship with the CEO of General Motors before you buy that new car. There are enough standards, laws and history for consumers to feel comfortable that they know more or less what to expect when they buy an automobile. Cars, although a relatively large purchase for the average consumer, have become a commodity. Licensing a major software application is a very different experience.

To be sure, there is commodity software, such as word processing and spreadsheet programs. (Most of us who have purchased the Microsoft Office Suite application do not have a personal relationship with Bill Gates). But most large, complex applications are not yet commodities. Their features and functions are highly variable, even among products that purport to do the same things. Thus what you buy is as much the company's vision and ongoing expertise as it is current features of the software.

Managing the vendor relationship once the EHR is embedded in your business processes is particularly complex. Once you have converted to an EHR you are, in a sense, sharing the management of your medical records with your vendor. Paper charts will quickly become outdated, leaving the EHR as the only effective source of clinical information. And whether you buy the EHR as a service (e.g., from an Application Service Provider—ASP), or contract to run the software onsite, there will be certain aspects of the system that will be beyond your control, e.g., system response time. For those issues, your vendor will be your only source of support. Having a partner that will respond to your issues, help resolve your problems and listen to your ideas is essential to your organization's success.

What Makes a Good Client-Vendor Relationship?

Companies, like people, have different personalities and styles. Finding a company that is compatible culturally, shares a common vision with you and, of course, has a product that meets your functional needs will give you a good chance at a long lasting, successful relationship. The nature of the relationship and the value proposition will likely be different depending on your organization's size and the scope of the implementation. Here are some suggestions that may help you to have a successful relationship with your vendor. We use all of them to one degree or another.

Get to Know the Company and Its Culture

Before you sign a contract, take the time to visit the company headquarters. Talk to as many people as you can, not just the CEO or department heads. Ask to talk to some of the software developers and engineers. Have a casual conversation with people in the hallway, if possible. What's the general feel you get walking around the company? What is the work environment like for the employees? Do people seem engaged and enthusiastic? What is the company's management style and philosophy? How do they find and keep good talent? What parts of the business do they seem to emphasize–marketing, development, testing, or implementation? Beware the software company that has more marketing staff than developers.

Understand the Business Model and What Drives the Company's Revenues

Most software companies rely on support fees to fund not only support, but ongoing development as well. Companies may sell you their product at a rock-bottom price and then charge higher-than-average maintenance fees. Make sure you understand the built-in escalation process for increasing costs over time. Tying increases to an external benchmark such as the consumer price index (CPI) is useful, if you can get your vendor to agree. In general software maintenance as a percentage of sales price has been rising steadily over the past several years and now ranges from 18% to 24%. In essence, you are repurchasing the application software every five years. Some vendors include major new releases of their software as part of the support cost, but others do not. Some charge a fee for every technical support call. Know what you will get for your support dollars.

If you are purchasing the system as a turnkey service (i.e., not running the system on site), it will be important for you understand the upgrade model, since the timing of upgrades (both hardware and software) may be out of your control.

As important as not paying too much for support is not paying too little. You are investing in a long-term relationship to manage one of your organization's most valuable assets. You need a partner that's going to be around for a while. Many CDOs have had to abandon an EHR project because the vendor underestimated their costs and went bankrupt.

Finally, it is important to understand the vendor's finances. Are they publicly held, and thus responsible to their investors and to Wall Street? This is not necessarily a negative, but will be important in understanding what influences the company's business strategy. What is their governance model? How much influence does a board of directors or other governing body exert on day-to-day operations? How much does the company's vision and ongoing success depend on its CEO or any other single individual?

Understand the Company's Long-Term Vision and Strategy

As much as anything, buying an EHR is buying into a vendor's vision and strategy. Most companies articulate a vision for their organization that goes far beyond where their products are presently. While plans for future development are often overly ambitious, understanding what markets or services a company is trying to move into over a two- to five-year horizon can be helpful in developing your own long-term plan. And, since no vendor can supply all the applications required in a complex healthcare organization, knowing what areas the vendor is planning to concentrate on can help you put together a comprehensive plan that includes systems from other sources.

Knowing the history of a company can give you insight into how successful they will be in future initiatives. Most EHR vendors started with patient accounting or clinical ancillary systems (e.g., lab). Where a company started may influence some of the strengths and weaknesses of their EHR. It is important to understand if their expertise has moved beyond these areas, since development of a functional EHR requires a broad understanding of all aspects of healthcare processes.

Identify Areas That Are Mutually Beneficial

Besides acting as a revenue source for the vendor, identify the value that you bring to the client-vendor relationship. Many vendors look to their best customers to provide input regarding new software functions, testing of new applications, and site visits for potential customers. Agreeing to be more than just a user of a company's product is one way to contribute to the relationship (and perhaps lower your support costs or have more direct input into product development).

Talk to and Visit Other Customers

Talking to existing customers can give you valuable insight into what a company is like to deal with. Keep in mind that the sites that vendors will take you to see will by definition be sites that are happy with the vendor. Request time alone with the host site representatives, and ask the vendor to disclose any reimbursement they are providing to the host for the visit. If possible, get a current client list and conduct additional interviews by telephone (without the vendor's involvement).

Take the Time to Develop a Good Contract

Contract negotiations can be tedious, but during the give and take of the negotiations you will learn a lot about the vendor and how they view their customers. Clarifying your mutual obligations will lay the foundation for a successful partnership. In addition, should the relationship sour, a well-crafted contract will protect your organization, particularly by guaranteeing your right to continue to use the software.

Here are some topics to agree on during contract negotiations:

Know Your Right to Use the Software

Particularly if you have a complex organizational structure, defining how, where and by whom the software can be used is important to avoid breaching the provisions of a contract. Is offering the use of the EHR to community physicians an important part of your business strategy? If so, you will want to make sure your vendor will support this both technically and legally. Even if you are a relatively small organization, you want to be sure that you have the right to use the software where and when you need it (e.g., in multiple physician offices, in affiliated facilities, or from home).

Understand the Maintenance Requirements for Your System

Some vendors will only allow use of the software as long you contract with them for maintenance. Having a maintenance contract for software of this nature may seem like a no-brainer, but consider what may happen when a system is at the end of its useful life. You may want the option to drop maintenance at some time in the future if you decide to replace the EHR. Some vendors will allow you to continue to run their systems without a maintenance contract in place, but charge hefty penalties if you later change your mind and want to reinstate the maintenance agreement. Make sure you understand what factors will affect maintenance prices.

Understand Your Obligation to Keep the Software Current

Contracts often stipulate how many release levels (i.e., versions of the software) the vendor will support. Upgrades can become complex and time-consuming once an EHR is in round-the-clock use. Consider contract language that protects you from having to accept an upgrade if you discover significant gaps in software function or stability.

Understand What Happens If the Company Goes Out of Business or is Acquired

Software companies and their products are often acquired by competitors solely to acquire market share. Then they discontinue the product—a process known as "sun-setting". You need to know what your rights are in this situation. Vendors will sometimes agree to put their source code (i.e., software programs) in escrow to be provided to the customer should they become insolvent. Vendors who discontinue support for an application generally offer incentives to customers who convert to their preferred products. Keep in mind, however, that an EHR conversion will be difficult and carry with it substantial risk. And, since all of these systems are relatively new, you can expect that there will be almost no conversion experience to draw upon.

Understand the Remedies Available to You for System Malfunctions, Software Bugs and Missing Software Functions

Problems will inevitably crop up during the implementation and operation of the system. How these are addressed, perhaps more than any other facet of the client-vendor partnership, defines the value of the relationship. Understand how a problem is reported, how it is escalated if necessary and how the solution is communicated back to you. The middle of a crisis is not the time to pull out the contract to see how the problem escalation process is supposed to work.

How to Keep Your Partner's Attention

Most vendors have a wide range of relationships with their customers, largely driven by how much effort each party puts into the relationship. Involvement in activities that add value to both parties is key. Although time-consuming, active participation in users groups, focus groups, advisory councils, special interest groups, site visits, etc. will go a long way toward capturing and keeping your partner's attention. In the end, time spent in this way will give you more influence on the development of the EHR and better support. Below are some specific thoughts regarding the different approaches we use to keep the vendor relationships positive.

Site Visits

Most vendors use site visits at some point in the sales cycle, to show what the software can do in a real-world setting. Since there is no substitute for this, vendors are generally willing to give special consideration to customers that are willing to take the time and effort to host potential customers. Many vendors will offer discounts on maintenance fees or other incentives as a way to compensate sites for the time and effort involved. Host sites also benefit from interaction with different organizations, in particular from discussions of workflow, processes and business strategy. Whether the potential client signs with the vendor, or not, there is value in interacting with peer organizations.

Users Groups

Most vendors have active users groups that meet at least annually. These meetings generally have three main objectives: (1) to serve as a platform for the vendor to showcase new products and new software functions, (2) to allow customers to present projects and accomplishments using the vendor's system, and (3) to provide feedback to the vendor regarding new functions that your organization needs. UGMs also provide a forum for customers to network and discuss common concerns and approaches to problems. Many large vendors also sponsor local or regional users groups that meet several times throughout the year. Vendors use these meetings to prioritize software change requests, as well as providing the same networking opportunity as the national meetings. Active participation in users groups is an excellent way to provide ongoing input to the vendor's development process.

Focus Groups, Advisory Councils, and Special Interest Groups

In addition to users groups, some vendors sponsor smaller gatherings with more focused agendas. These gatherings are often organized by role, such as physician groups or scheduling groups. These meetings often exert the most direct effect on product development.

Executive Meetings

Periodically it is good idea to have top management from each of the partner organizations get together to discuss the state of the relationship. This can include presentations of each party's strategies, current environment, needs and a general discussion of how well (or not) things are going. This reinforces the partnership and is an opportunity for executive leadership to work out any high-level concerns or issues. These meetings will also help your organization's IT and executive leadership to refine your IT strategies.

Beta Site Participation

Being a beta test site for new software can serve as a good mechanism for providing direct input into new system features and functions. Unfortunately, it can also be very disruptive to your operation, since beta code by its nature is unstable and prone to bugs. Organizations that act as test sites for vendor software generally do so at their own risk. Also, most vendors require a formal agreement to insure that sufficient testing is done to test all the new features and functions of the application. This means dedicating sufficient resources to comply. Since the EHR is such a critical part of clinical operations, testing new software should be done with caution. A separate environment where extensive off-line tests can be performed before putting new code into production works best.

The general theme of all of these techniques is to be proactive—stay involved in the forums that keep you connected to your vendor. Contacting your partner only when you want something or have a problem is not the best way to build a relationship, or keep the vendor focused on your account.

Requesting System Modifications and Customizations

Every system can stand to be improved. Vendors are continually bombarded with requests for expanded functions and new features. Most have methods for vetting ideas from their customers, so that they can be incorporated into general releases (rather than delivered as custom software to a particular site). While having the vendor write custom computer code specifically for your organization is sometimes unavoidable, use this option only as a last resort. Our experience has been that using custom code from the vendor (or worse, writing it yourself) makes the upgrade process extremely complex, and in some cases almost unmanageable. Working with the vendor to get the features you want incorporated into the base software by working with fellow customers is usually the most efficient method to get the functions you want. Over time, custom software drives up the cost of the system due to the extensive testing required for every upgrade. It may make your system unstable. Some vendors do give you the ability to add code at certain specific points within their applications with the assurance that they will not be affected by software upgrades. This reduces the costs of adding custom code, but it still adds complexity to system support, particularly upgrade testing.

Managing Multiple Vendors

Most healthcare organizations do not have the luxury of dealing with just one vendor for all their software needs. The amount of effort and complexity involved in coordinating multiple vendors will depend on the size and complexity of your organization. But even a single physician's practice usually has external as well as internal sources of information, many of which will need to be incorporated into the EHR. And the EHR, even assuming it is purchased or leased from a single vendor, contains components from various companies, such as lists of medicines or diagnostic codes. Over the years, we have coordinated the efforts of many vendors to insure that the systems we install work as seamlessly as possible. Here are some practices that we have found useful:

EHR Vendor

The EHR that you acquire (assuming you run the system on-site) will have at a minimum the following three components: (1) the hardware and operating system, (2) the database system, and (3) the application software. Usually EHR vendors try to shield their customers from having to deal extensively with the first two components of the system. This can be effective in small organizations that have little complexity. For midsize or large organizations (i.e., those having hundreds or thousands of users), establishing a relationship with the main hardware and database provider can make overall system support easier. Understanding how the components work together can decrease troubleshooting time, optimize the testing process and make capacity planning and upgrade planning easier. This can be as simple as periodic meetings with the EHR vendor and the other parties where you learn what is being planned for upcoming releases and what problems and issues have been encountered at other sites.

Other Partners

Because your EHR becomes the central repository for clinical data, most organizations must deal with interfaces. Laboratory data, transcribed documents and insurance information are just a few examples of systems that are typically interfaced with the EHR. In most mid- to large-sized CDOs, departmental systems for lab, radiology, pharmacy and cardiology all come from different vendors. Coordinating the interfaces to and from these systems to your EHR mainly falls to you. While the technical challenge is significant, you will also face the challenge of keeping each vendor's proprietary intellectual property secure, while at the same time integrating your data and their software functions into a seamless flow.

Summary

With the plethora of companies and systems to choose from, selecting and managing a partner can be a challenge. Trust is an important factor in a successful partnership, but blind trust can lead to misunderstandings and failed relationships. Spend time getting to know your vendor before signing a contract. Work with the vendor and their products to bring value to the partnership, and your organization will receive more from your partner in return.

Part Three
Implementation

14
Phased Implementation

Linda M. Culp, Jean A. Adams, Janet S. Byron, and
Elizabeth A. Boyer

Phased implementation is the stepwise introduction of EHR functionality through a series of phases, each with its own analysis, training, and go-live schedule. A phased approach spreads the users' learning over time, producing several manageable peaks in cognitive load. (Figure 14.1) This reduces training needs and the productivity loss typically associated with EHR implementation.

We learned phased implementation in the school of hard knocks, as we implemented the first few practices with the "Big Bang". This method combined the implementation of the scheduling application, all the functions of the EHR, and re-designed workflows in one project. Support staff, nursing personnel, and providers finished eight hours of training on patient scheduling and 24 hours of EHR training on a Friday. On the following Monday, the practice's front desk staff began using the new electronic patient scheduling and registration systems. At the same time, clinicians began placing orders and documenting the visit (e.g., vital signs, history and physical, orders, level of service) in the EHR. This "Big Bang"—despite careful planning, adequate implementation team staffing, and physician schedules that were reduced by 50% for go-live, resulted in:

- Practice chaos: Clerical staff, nurses, and providers' work slowed almost to a stop. This was exacerbated by the fact that Monday is the busiest day for most primary-care practices.
- Inability to absorb and retain training.
- Substantial productivity losses. Even with schedules reduced by half, the practices were unable to keep up with patient volumes.
- Need for a dress rehearsal: Practices had no alternative but to come in during off hours (i.e., evenings and weekends) to practice the new workflows and the use of the software. Family members served as "patients" while physicians and staff practiced using the EHR.

The chaos produced by the "Big Bang" required us to change our approach. We began by implementing the scheduling and registration applications throughout the organization before we resumed the EHR implementation. Then we divided the EHR implementation into three phases: (1) test results viewing, transcription authentication, and e-messaging; (2) electronic results distribution; and (3) order entry and visit documentation. Finally, we streamlined training (see Chapter 8) into two two-hour sessions, tailored to specific user needs.

Stabilizing the scheduling and patient registration software and workflows prior to the EHR implementation produced several benefits:

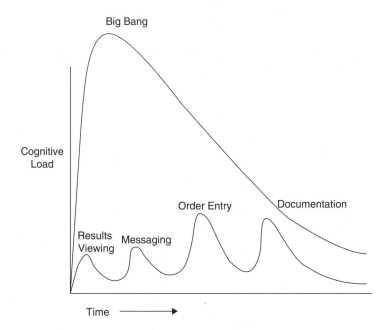

FIGURE 14.1. Managing cognitive load with phased implementation.

- When the EHR was implemented, clerical workers were able to process patients rapidly, eliminating one set of workflow problems.
- Electronic check-in made using the EHR easier for nurses and physicians, because they could pick patients from schedules rather than searching for them in the database.
- Clerical workers were able to help the clinicians learn EHR skills.
- The scheduling and registration systems produced lists of patients scheduled for appointments during the first few weeks of go-live. This allowed us to abstract their charts in preparation for go-live. The availability of medical histories, problem lists, and medication lists in the EHR made the critical first weeks after go-live far easier for clinicians.

Phase 1: Access to Test Results and Transcribed Documents

Viewing test results in the EHR requires little training since its main effect is to make a familiar workflow easier. One-hour classroom sessions with or without computer-based training were all that most users needed. We implemented the viewing function for 600 physicians in 70 practice sites in six-months.

Site Preparation

This phase required the placement of a PC in every outpatient exam room. Since most of these rooms had limited space already, the monitor often took up most of the desktop. Mitigating this space crunch required the cooperation of the practice's operations, office support, nursing, and physician staffs (along with the IT technical team) in a device placement walkthrough. During the first walk-through the team balanced the need for easily available PCs and printers (for order requisitions and prescriptions) with other needs. A second walk-through added representatives from facilities management, who identified renovation needs, such as additional electrical outlets and network cabling. The lead nurse and physician in each site authorized the final placement plan.

Chart Abstraction

Pre-populating the EHR with basic patient information abstracted from the paper chart contributes powerfully to the success of this first phase. As Clem MacDonald (one of the most experienced and thoughtful developers of EHRs) says, "Physicians love to get data. They hate to give data." (1). This is especially true of new users, who are frequently overloaded with the need to remember a new ID and password, new workflows, and new software skills—all while caring for patients. Abstracting provides the basic information users need to interpret test results, decreasing the need to refer to the paper chart. Chart abstraction also provides effective EHR training. We provide our physicians with a two-sided summary sheet for documenting patient identifiers, allergies, problems (with comments), medicines, and history of disease preventive care. Completing this form and pre-populating patients' electronic records with the data is an effective way for physicians to prepare for go-live.

Chart abstraction can be organized in various ways. We have used these methods in different settings. Reports from other organizations indicate successful use of others. The key to success is matching the method to resource availability and to the working style of each practice.

One method is to require physicians to abstract the paper charts of patients they are scheduled to see in the first month after go-live and then enter the data into the EHR. With this method, the abstracter is the person best able to abstract the chart accurately and succinctly. It also gives providers effective, low stress practice using the EHR. One problem with this approach, however, is that most physicians are worse at data input than less expensive clerical workers. This will make the approach resource-expensive if providers are paid for large-scale chart abstraction. Not many physicians will use their free time for abstracting charts.

A second method is to pay dedicated personnel to do both chart abstraction and data entry. In most organizations, these are nurses—whose clinical training and experience is usually considered necessary for safe and effective abstraction. This approach has the virtue of predictable performance and known costs. However, abstraction by nurses is likely to be less clinically precise than if the patient's physician performs the abstraction. Nurses also make expensive data entry personnel.

A final method is to provide clerical data input for all chart abstractions that physicians complete before go-live. This approach motivates physicians to make their unique contribution in time for it to be effective and provides cost-effective data entry. The abstraction forms mentioned above help physicians abstract completely and efficiently (see Appendix 10).

Scanning

Abstracting charts alerted us to the large volumes of clinically relevant documents that would not be incorporated electronically (as codified data) into the EHR (e.g., pulmonary function tests and EKG results). Scanning provides a valuable way to include these reports. However, scanning has several drawbacks. Unless it is performed selectively, it can produce masses of information within which it is impossible to search efficiently. Even when performed selectively, scanning produces records that cannot be stored in the same location (in our EHR) as electronically transferred reports. For example, a scanned EKG must be filed under "scanned documents," rather than with electronically transferred EKG's. If scanning is used as a substitute for paper chart abstraction, the allergy lists, problem list and medicine lists (whose fields must be filled with codified data (e.g., "diabetes with neurological manifestations, 250.62") will remain empty. For this reason, scanning should be used to store documents for occasional reference, while abstraction and electronic data entry should be used to enter data that clinicians will need on a regular basis. For example, a pulmonary function test, if scanned into the chart, should still be summarized on the problem list, e.g., "shortness of breath: PFTs nl, 5/04."

Initially, we provided each practice with a scanner, but without dedicated personnel and high-speed scanners, capacity never kept pace with demand. By the time we switched to centralized scanning, our practices had a backlog of nearly 1.4 million pages waiting to be scanned. Centralized scanning, with high-speed scanners, enabled us to eliminate the backlog, provided access to every scanned document throughout the system (by way of storage on a central server), and reduced total scanning costs from $0.62 per page to $0.23 (with a turnaround time of 24 hours).

Phase 2: Electronic Results Distribution, Transcription Authentication, and E-Messaging

In this phase, test results and transcribed documents are sent to providers' inbaskets for review and electronic signature. Like the first phase, these added EHR functions make familiar workflows faster and more efficient than they have been in the past, particularly because of the remote access (including home access) they provide. Additional advantages include:

- Elimination of printing, distribution and filing of paper copies of test results and transcriptions
- Linking transcribed documents to the appropriate patient encounter (e.g., to a specific office visit)
- Electronic communication among clinicians linked to patient records

Along with results and transcription distribution, Phase 2 introduces electronic management of patients' medication renewal requests and other telephone messages. Since the EHR's messaging works like standard e-mail with a convenient link to the patient's record, it enables improved clinical communications with minimal learning (although new workflows for managing patient requests do require design and training).

This phase completed the EHR implementation for clerical personnel, who have a large role in triaging incoming messages and responding to patient requests. Nursing staff, whose work had been minimally affected by the first two phases, began to use the EHR more heavily in this phase for triaging patient requests and initiating the responses (e.g., entering prescriptions for providers to authenticate and release).

E-messaging creates the first opportunity to customize the EHR to the needs of specific practices. Customized lists of medications, diagnoses, and reasons for patient requests provide users with short pick-lists of frequently used items. For example, a pediatrics nurse typing "amox" sees the pediatric formulations and doses of amoxicillin, where a nurse in an internal medicine practice sees a different list that is appropriate for adults (see Table 15.1).

Benefits

The introduction of electronic inbaskets brings with it the opportunity to decrease the printing and filing (the expensive steps) of paper reports. After a new electronic system has been in place long enough to prove itself reliable and for clinicians to become used to using it (one to three months), we discontinue production of paper copies (with the concurrence of affected clinical and administrative leaders).

Training and Retraining

This phase provides a golden opportunity to review EHR use with physicians who have avoided using the EHR to this point, but begin to recognize the value (or inevitability) of EHR use.

Phase 3: Order Entry and Patient-Care Documentation

Although order entry and documentation began as two distinct phases, over time they became two aspects of a single implementation phase. This was prompted by the request of several practices to begin documentation at the same time as order entry. In most practices, Phases 1 and 2 had prepared users sufficiently that implementing order entry and documentation together was more efficient than doing them separately.

Preparation

The implementation of an EHR changes information access and the division of clinical labor. (Keen (2) provides a succinct, authoritative discussion.) For example, will nurses prepare drug renewals for physicians to authorize, or will physicians perform the entire process? Since these decisions can be disruptive, it is critical to involve all stakeholders in a transparent and accountable process of workflow development. Since different practices will answer the questions differently, we allow each practice considerable latitude in modifying workflows to reflect their unique circumstances.

The initial planning (or pre-kickoff) meeting includes operations managers, physician leaders, the Chief Medical Information Officer, a healthcare informatician, and IT project directors. It is held two weeks before the kick-off meeting, which is attended by the entire practice. The agenda for this two-hour pre-kickoff meeting includes:

- Implementation Scope: The operational needs and goals of the practice are elicited, with explicit attention given to ancillary services, specialized personnel, special-purpose software needs, and the facility's physical layout.
- Responsibilities Document (see Appendix 9): This document, jointly developed by the practice's leaders and the implementation team, details implementation steps, the respective responsibilities of the members of the practice implementation team for each step, and the project's timeline. Negotiation of the document's specific contents creates the mutual understanding necessary for a successful implementation.

- Timeline: A generic timeline is modified to meet the needs of the practice. For instance, implementation during the flu season should be avoided in primary-care practices. Similarly, national meetings can derail go-lives in specialty practices.
- Establishment of project teams
  - A project control team meets weekly to monitor the project's progress and make implementation decisions.
  - Providers from the practice and the projects' physician informatician meet regularly to develop efficiency tools such as note templates and order sets.
- Issue escalation: We identify a practice leader and an IT leader to whom the control team can escalate problems that it is unable to resolve. This process is rarely required, but invaluable when needed. (For an example, see the OB/Gyn case study in Chapter 16.)
- Training Schedule: The training needed by various user groups is reviewed to enable practice leaders to make scheduling and budgetary plans.
- Communications
  - A project binder, kept in a convenient location in each practice, records the implementation's progress. It contains meeting minutes, issues lists, workflows, and preference lists.
  - An EHR bulletin board (for posting meeting minutes, training session dates and times, and efficiency tips) helps to keep everyone informed of practice progress and training opportunities.

Kick-Off

The implementation kick-off meeting is scheduled by the practice for about two weeks after the pre-kickoff meeting. All practice personnel—clerical staff, nursing, residents, physician extenders and physicians—attend.

The agenda for the Kick-off Meetings includes the following elements:

- *The practice's role in the implementation:* Practice leaders (clinical and managerial) present the responsibilities document agreed upon at the pre-kick-off meeting. Each practice member receives a copy.
- *EHR Demonstration:* An informatician uses the EHR to document a complete patient encounter, using scenarios specific to that particular practice. In the first part of the demonstration, the informatician completes the encounter without interruption, allowing the clinicians to see how rapidly an encounter can be completed using well-designed, customized note templates and order sets. After this, the floor is opened to questions, with answers illustrated by repeating relevant parts of the demonstration. Areas in which the practice has the opportunity to develop customized tools are particularly emphasized.
- *Issues Identification:* Questions that the implementation team is not able to answer are included on the list of issues to be addressed during implementation analysis and workflow design.

Control Team

Hour-long implementation Control Team meetings are held weekly, with day, time and location selected by the clinic. The team's role is to identify issues, elicit input from the practice, plan resolutions, and communicate them to the practice. The Control Team is made up of scheduling and registration clerks, nurses, physicians, billing coders, and operations managers. The Implementation Team, along with practice leaders, creates the agenda, which is distributed along with minutes of the previous meeting. Control team members receive early training on the EHR and receive special ongoing EHR support.

Order Entry

Order entry requires more effort from the practice and individual clinicians than any of the earlier phases. One of the first tasks is the creation of customized pick lists of diagnoses, tests, procedures and drugs. One of the keys to creating effective lists is translating the sometimes confusing standard lists into language that is familiar to clinicians. To start the process, we compile preliminary lists of favorites from billing system and laboratory system records and previous implementations in similar practices. Almost every practice has a few clinicians who will edit these lists quickly and add items that are absent. (These lists also help identify diagnoses for which order sets may be most useful.)

Provider and nursing input into the EHR customization is best spread over two months. This two-month timeframe allows the team and the providers to focus on one or a few lists and order sets at a time. As a final check, the practice physician leaders, the practice manager, and billing department validate the appropriateness of the proposed preference lists and order sets.

Billing Support

Our physicians have become increasingly knowledgeable about appropriate billing methods over the last several years. Even so, electronic order entry provides an opportunity to document care more fully and bill more accurately. To take advantage of this opportunity, our billing department teaches providers a required class on the use of diagnoses and procedure codes, levels of service, and appropriate documentation for services. As is the case for EHR training in general, such courses focus on practice-appropriate scenarios. Implementation analysts attend these classes to understand how to use the EHR to support more accurate billing and to respond to provider's questions.

Using the EHR to support more accurate billing requires sustained the cooperation of implementation analysts, the practice's billing specialist, the practice manager, and clinicians. In weekly meetings, these participants identify scores of opportunities to customize the EHR and the standard workflows to improve practice performance. Many of the proposed customizations require the combined legal, safety, billing and medical education review provided by our healthcare-team integration committee (see Chapter 10). The presence of this committee allows implementation analysts to identify these often complex questions, refer them to the committee, and then implement the committee's decisions with a minimal effect on the project timeline.

The billing department's role extends to providing shadowing support at go-live. In addition, they perform post-implementation audits of documentation, orders, and billing codes to identify opportunities for additional training and for refining preference lists and order sets.

Documentation

In the documentation phase, users begin to enter clinical assessments and plans directly into the EHR. The EHR software makes it easy to build note templates and importable boilerplate that allow a skilled user to document a typical office visit by hitting only 20 to 30 keystrokes and typing several sentences. As with preference lists, the implementation team collects samples of the most commonly dictated or handwritten documents from the paper medical records. Armed with these samples, informaticians meet with the practice's domain expert (see chapter 9) to prioritize note templates and to identify their contents. After a tool is completed, the practice's other providers and the billing department review and comment on the template. After go-live, most practices' domain experts continue building the tools with only occasional assistance.

How to Push a Rope

Despite repeated reminders to the domain expert and careful coordination with physician leaders and practice managers, several domain experts were so late in providing content for tool-building (usually because the power of the tools is hard to comprehend before one uses the EHR, and because some practice leaders provided little support or encouragement) that the success of the documentation phase was at risk. Our response was to have a physician informatician use written and transcribed notes to create note templates (or order sets) and then ask users for feedback. Several of the domain experts we approached in this way became active tool builders when they saw the effectiveness of the tools in practice.

Technical Support

Phased implementation requires frequent changes in the system settings that determine access to the EHR functions (e.g., read-only, messaging, order entry). Careful coordination assures that these changes are implemented for each user at the appropriate times. The analyst responsible for the system setting worked on-site in each practice during the first few days of go-live so that they could provide immediate responses to requests for set-up changes. Few changes were needed, but having the analyst immediately available avoided user frustration and allowed them to focus on learning new workflows and software functions.

Pre-Go-Live Anxiety

Two weeks before order entry go-live, almost every practice expressed significant anxiety about its ability to use the EHR in daily practice. Some formally requested that the go-live be delayed. After we became aware of this pattern, the CMIO scheduled a pre-go-live meeting with each practice's lead physician two weeks before implementation. The CMIO reviewed the progress of the implementation and the successes of other similar practices. He also passed the leader's concerns to the implementation teams for resolution. These meetings produced a significant improvement in the morale of most practices as they approached go-live. There were no further requests for postponement.

Summary

The core principle of phased implementation is simply to begin with the least disruptive, most useful EHR functions, and then move to increasingly demanding functions as users increase their skills and see the benefits of an EHR. This approach has enabled us to move 4,000 users (including 600 physicians) to full EHR use with a minimum of disruption to patient care or practice efficiency.

References

1. McDonald C. The Regenstrief Medical Record System: 30 years of learning. AMIA Fall Symposium; Washington, DC: AMIA; 2001.
2. Keen PGW. Information systems and organizational change. *Comm ACM* 1981;24:24.

15
Optimizing Primary-Care Practices

ELLIE E. HENRY

Optimizing the EHR to support desired workflows is critical to user acceptance and to practice efficiency. Optimization requires understanding your current workflows and how they can be made more efficient with an EHR. This chapter will explain key steps to optimizing primary-care practice efficiency—prior to, during, and after go-live. (See Chapter 14 for our basic implementation methods.)

Workflows

The first step is to understand in detail the functions performed by your EHR software. The use of some of these will be critical to the EHR's effectiveness. Others will be optional; this is a critical distinction. Visiting other organizations that use the EHR and conducting phone interviews will help you understand the choices of functions, set-up requirements, and other implementation issues you will need to address.

Once you have a basic understanding of the EHR software, you will need to analyze and document your current workflows (see Chapter 5). The box below contains an example of workflow documentation:

Telephone Message:

1. Front office staff takes the message.
2. The paper chart is pulled and the message attached.
3. The chart is placed in the appropriate nurse's in-basket
4. The nurse reviews the message and responds or brings the chart to a provider.
5. If necessary, the provider reviews the message, documents the response and places the chart in the out-basket (or walks the chart to a nurse).
6. The nurse calls the patient with the response and documents the call in the chart.
7. The nurse returns the chart to the front office.
8. The front office staff files the chart.

This detailed analysis is needed for every major workflow in the practice (e.g., patient registration, phone calls, patient visits, patient check-out). After workflows are documented, they need to be verified by clinical leaders and practice managers. The leaders then decide which actions or steps will be eliminated, changed, or added, and which will remain the same.

In the telephone message example, the steps in bold represent those that were eliminated. The normal font represents steps that remained the same. (Note that implementing the EHR reduced the number of steps from eight to four).

1. The front office staff takes the message (and forwards it to a nurse's electronic in-basket).
2. **The paper chart is pulled and the message attached.**
3. **The chart is placed in the appropriate nurse in-basket.**
4. The nurse reviews the message and responds or forwards the message to a provider.
5. If necessary, the provider reviews the message, documents the response in the EHR and forwards the message (electronically) to the nurse pool.
6. A nurse calls the patient with the response, and documents the call in the EHR, and closes the encounter.
7. **The nurse returns the chart to the front office staff.**
8. **The front office staff person files the chart.**

Once you have eliminated unnecessary steps, focus on the steps that will not be eliminated but should change. Enlist all participants in the workflow to think about how the EHR can enable improvement in each remaining step of the process. Design new steps that are maximally efficient for all participants and that match each participant's mental model of the process as closely as possible. This matching will make the new process appear intuitive, with the effect that participants will execute the new process with less training, less effort, and fewer errors.

Any EHR project will change your organization. Your design team must consider whether each proposed change is likely to create benefits large enough to justify the effort required to put it into effect. In our experience, EHR users become more interested in using the EHR as a change tool after it is in use for six to twelve months. This makes it feasible to defer some workflow changes from the initial implementation project to ongoing workflow improvement efforts.

Preference Lists

A preference list is a short (usually less than 20 items) list of diagnoses, medications, or orders that the user first sees after typing a word or phrase into an appropriate search field. The preference list for each practice should include the most common diagnoses and procedural codes (which your billing and revenue staff or business manager can provide) and the most commonly prescribed doses and regimens of medications (see Table 15.1). To be effective, these preference lists should include the information needed to document about 80% of patient visits, while remaining short enough for fast searching and selection.

As new medications are approved, new diagnoses added, and new procedures performed, preference lists will need to be updated. Users will also identify many diagnoses and procedures that they cannot find in ICD-9 and CPT-4 (e.g., Schatzki's ring). In our EHR, creating synonyms for these missing or hard to find diagnoses and procedures is easy. The larger challenge is making it easy for users to inform the production support team about synonyms they need. When a clinician becomes aware of a

TABLE 15.1. Drug Preference Lists.

When a user types "amox" into the orders field, they see one of these two lists, depending on whether the user cares for adults or children. (Family practitioners see a list that combines the two). Without customized preference lists, every user would see 48 formulations and regimens of amoxicillin.

Adult Medicine			
Amoxicillin 250 mg tab	Take one pill 3 times a day for 10 days	Dispense #30	Refill #0
Amoxicillin 500 mg tab	Take one pill 3 times a day for 10 days	Dispense #30	Refill #0
Pediatrics			
Amoxicillin 250 mg/5 cc liquid	One teaspoon 3 times a day for 10 days	Dispense #150 cc	Refill #0
Amoxicillin 250 mg Chewable	One pill 3 times a day for 10 days	Dispense #30	Refill #0

need for a new synonym, she is usually seeing patients—and too busy to take the time to call the Help Desk or even to send an e-mail. It can be useful to have paper forms placed under the computer keyboard in exam rooms and physician offices so that they are available for requesting new synonyms, although the forms are hard to keep available and hard to collect. Most preference list requests come from domain experts, super-users, and practice managers (see Chapter 9)—or come up in re-training sessions.

Charting Tools

Complete, focused, timely documentation of clinical observations is fundamental to creating useful patient records (on paper or in an EHR). Efficient note templates and other charting tools can make capture of standardized data feasible, while retaining the flexibility of free-text entry. See below an example of a template for documenting the history and examination of a patient with new onset, benign new-onset low back pain.

Template for Low Back Pain

The patient notes new low back pain. There is no personal history of cancer, trauma, or long-term steroid use. The patient has noted no fever, unexplained weight loss, urinary retention, saddle anesthesia, fecal incontinence, sciatica, or bone pain.

On exam, the lungs are clear to auscultation and percussion, {the breasts are normal} {the prostate is without nodules}. There is no spinal tenderness to percussion. Both ipsilateral straight leg raising and crossed straight leg raising are negative. There is no ankle dorsiflexion, nor great toe extensor weakness.

***

{Early lumbar X-ray is not indicated when all of the above are negative.

Deyo, R. A., J. Rainville, et al. (1992). The rational clinical examination: what can the history and physical examination tell us about low back pain?" JAMA 268(6): 760–765.

Validated by Performance Improvement and Billing, April 2003.}
Plan:
{Ibuprofen 400 mg PO TID}
{Lorazepam 0.5 mg PO qHS}
{Activity ad lib}
{Return to Clinic 1 month}

The note can be completed with six keyboard strokes. It reminds the user of the criteria from Deyo's landmark study (1), which, if all negative, identify patients who do not require diagnostic imaging and who have a 90% likelihood of recovery in one month, if they are active as tolerated and take pain medicine as needed. It also gives the user the option of adding whatever free text is appropriate, at the triple asterisk prompt. The elements in curly braces can be removed or accepted with a single keystroke. Most users leave them to document their decision-making.

A robust collection of note templates available at go-live enables users to document directly into the EHR—improving the quality of notes and saving transcription costs without suffering productivity losses. Begin by developing note templates and associated order sets for the most common problems and visit types (e.g., annual physicals). As users become comfortable with the EHR (usually three to six months after go-live), enlist users (i.e., Domain Experts) in each practice to receive training and EHR team support to enable them to continue to build charting and other tools for their workgroup. We bring these clinical domain experts together every two months for an all day tool-building workshop. They bring content for note templates and order sets from their practices and build the tools with IT and billing department support. (See Chapter 9.)

Chart Abstraction

Abstracting pertinent patient information from the paper medical record and entering it into the EHR provides critical preparation for go-live. The availability of relevant patient information during the first patient visits will make users' initial experience with the EHR more efficient and satisfactory. Abstracting also provides hands-on practice in entering information into the EHR, increasing users' skills at reading EHR screens and entering information. (See Chapter 14 for details)

Patient Acceptance

In addition to improving patient safety, the EHR can improve patients' experience of your organization. Our own research and that of others (2) suggests that patients appreciate the use of computers during office visits.

We have used two main strategies to achieve this satisfaction. First, we informed patients ahead of time that we were transitioning to the use of computerized records.

We mailed informational letters, placed posters and brochures in waiting areas and exam rooms, and used the news media (particularly newspapers) to spread the word. Patients contacted us (largely face-to-face, but also by phone) with questions and concerns. These were mostly related to the security of the information in the EHR and who would be able to see the information. The clinical front desk staff handled most of these questions, but some were triaged to nurses and physicians, based on patient need. Second, we collaborated with the Bayer Institute to train physicians on ways to make the EHR a positive part of a patient's office visit.

Post-Implementation Support

Extensive post-go-live support is critical to a successful implementation (3). In primary-care practices, we find that a combination of shadow support and super-users is most effective. We normally provide shadow training for two weeks after go-live. Infrequently, we extend shadowing to meet the needs of physicians who are infrequently in the clinics and others who have difficulty using the EHR. Close coordination between shadow trainers and super-users provides ongoing user training and support after shadow training ends.

Go-live is a critical step in EHR implementation. However, rather than marking the end of your work, it marks the beginning of the next phase—several years of enhancing the EHR system and the skills of your EHR users. There are several ways to do this. One is to make the EHR a standing agenda item at practice staff meetings, addressing usability needs, missing software functions, and opportunities to support improved workflows.

It is difficult to assign resources to post-implementation training while your teams are in the midst of an aggressive EHR rollout schedule. However, it is our experience (and the experience of many other organizations) that, when we go back even into clinics that are successfully using the EHR, we find substantial opportunities to improve the EHR to fit improved workflows. For this reason, we have increased the resources devoted to post-go-live training over time, developing various methods of providing post-live training to our primary care practices.

Tips and Tricks

We publish concise, practical EHR tips via e-messaging and on an internal Web site (See Box below.)

Tips and Tricks

When in the charting screen, you can review old encounters easily by using the COPY PREVIOUS button. This allows you to copy and paste old notes into the current encounter. The button is located above the charting documentation area on the charting screen.

We send these tips on an irregular schedule—about every two weeks. We limit the number of tips to three per message. Many users find them helpful.

EHR Workshops for Providers and Support Staff

Instructor-led, hands-on workshops allow time for one-on-one instruction. In our experience, a class size of two provides the optimal educational experience. Based on participants' feedback and the impacts on individual and practice productivity, we believe that the benefits of these workshops justify their cost. We also believe that they would remain highly effective with a maximum of five to six participants.

The workshop curriculum is focused on efficient use of the EHR—for example, through keyboard shortcuts and use of note templates and order sets. Over time, we have developed two distinct curricula—one for providers, the other for clinical support staff. This allows for a more focused, role-specific curriculum and more productive sharing of insights among learners.

Physicians, mid-level providers, and nursing staff who attend the four-hour introductory workshop earn four hours of professional education credit, making it easier for them to justify their time away from patient care.

Users' group meetings are another effective venue for post-implementation training. (See Chapter 8.)

Webcasting

Webcasting allows participants to view the convener's computer screen during a telephone conference call, while they converse via telephone. The technology allows the participants to develop improved workflows and EHR tools collaboratively. The convener reports the group's work products to practice leaders for validation and to the EHR production-support team for implementation.

Post-Implementation Training Reviews

Most users need a few months to integrate the basic functions of the EHR into their workflows. For this reason, few clinics are ready for post-implementation training before three months following go-live. We attempt to schedule sessions at three months, six months, and one year post-go-live. To ensure maximum relevance, the post-implementation training team (2.0 FTEs) and the billing department review the EHR of 30 of the practice's patients, along with the practice's preference lists. They interview clinical and administrative staff to identify discrepancies between planned and actual workflows and areas of user confusion and dissatisfaction.

Practices need one to two months' advance notice of post-live training sessions to give them time to prepare questions and to suggest changes to the system build (e.g., new diagnoses to be added to the preference lists). Because practice leaders have neither the time nor the experience to conduct such reviews, EHR team members staff the reviews under the joint leadership of practice managers and an IT director.

Communication

Notifying users and managers about system downtimes, upgrades, and other changes to the EHR is critical for practice efficiency. To be useful, communications must be short and free of IT jargon. They must tell users what they need to know and nothing more. For example, they need to know what services will be unavailable and for how long, what the alternative sources of information are, and whom to call with questions. To make the task of creating and reading these messages more efficient and error-free, develop a template for creating them (see Box below).

Example Message

The EHR will be unavailable this Saturday, January 10, from 6:00 PM to 8:00 PM for a system upgrade.

During the downtime, read-only access to information entered into the EHR before the beginning of the downtime (that is, the shadow EHR) will continue to be available, but it will not be updated after 6:00 PM.

To access the EHR during the downtime, click on the "EHR Shadow" icon on the desktop. When the downtime is over, it will take approximately 30 minutes for all the results that were completed during the downtime to file into the EHR.

The communications plan for unscheduled downtimes will require back-up communication channels. Telephone calls to practices, overhead paging, Help Desk automated replies, and personally delivered messages may all be needed, depending on the extent of the downtime.

Training Reference Materials

Your organization's Intranet is an efficient means of providing support materials—including training manuals, workflow charts, and frequently asked questions. Of course, most users will not remember that these materials exist (or be able to find them if they do remember). One effective method of reminding users is to send an e-message (e.g., Tips and Tricks) with a link to the more extensive information included. We also provide EHR System-Build Change order forms (e.g., for requesting a new diagnosis synonym) and EHR Access Request forms on our Intranet. Another effective method (if desktop space is available) is to have an "EHR Help" icon on the desktop of all clinical computers.

Home Access

Home access to the EHR does not necessarily make primary-care physicians more efficient, but it does give them flexibility in their work, which many value highly. Some like to complete documentation at home, allowing them to eat dinner with their families first. Others have come to regard access to the EHR as necessary when they are on-call or attending at other hospitals. Some want to review a patient's record as they prepare to come to the hospital for a consult.

Loaner Laptops

Many primary-care practices provide loaner laptops for physicians and mid-level providers to take with them when they are on-call or attending conferences. This allows them to provide continuity of care while away from the office.

Laptop software is limited to the EHR, e-mail, and Internet access. Users cannot save documents to the hard drive, but are able to e-mail documents to themselves for later storage.

Other providers use their own computers at home. (See Chapter 4.)

Summary

Optimizing the use of the EHR for primary-care practices is an iterative process. It begins with a cooperative effort by clinicians, administrators, and EHR teams to build the EHR so that it is capable of supporting desired workflows. The same partnership then needs to review each practice regularly to identify further usability, workflow improvement, and training opportunities.

References

1. Deyo RA, Rainville J, Kent D. The rational clinical examination: what can the history and physical examination tell us about low back pain? *JAMA* 1992;268(6):760–765.
2. Anderson J, Kaplan B. Evaluating the impact of health care information systems. AMIA Annual Symposium. 2001; Washington, DC: AMIA; 2001.
3. Ash JS, Stavri PZ, Kuperman GJ. A consensus statement on considerations for a successful CPOE implementation. *J Am Med Informatics* 2003;10:229–234.

16
Optimizing Specialty Practices

LINDA M. CULP

Many organizations settle for "plain vanilla" implementations (e.g., identical note templates and order sets) for all their primary and specialty care practices, despite the different workflows and information management needs of different practices. This approach contributes to some outright implementation failures and many missed opportunities for efficiency and quality improvement.

The first task of the implementation team is to analyze practice workflows and understand the commonalities and differences between various practices. This knowledge enables the team to create a standardized, efficient implementation process that meets each practice's unique needs. This chapter builds on Chapter 14 and Chapter 15, providing details on implementing this standardized process to produce effective specialty practice implementations

---

Specialty Care and Customization: A Caveat

Every practice we have implemented had special customization needs. This was true for each of our 42 primary-care practices, as well as our specialty practices. What is different about specialty practices is the degree of variation among them and the large numbers of specialties to be implemented (about 70 in our system).

We developed many of the principles and methods presented in this chapter for primary-care practices. We now apply them to new implementations of both primary and specialty care practices.

Specialty-Practice Complexities

Collaborative Care

Phased implementation of hospital-based specialty practices can involve intricacies not encountered in freestanding practices:

- The use of a single, shared paper medical record requires that charts are pulled for each patient visit until every practice has gone live on the EHR (in case a paper-based provider has added a note to the chart).

- Multispecialty clinics have providers that rotate to various sites and share support staff. This requires painstaking integration of scheduling, patient registration, documentation, test ordering, test results distribution, and billing.
- Complex patients require collaborative care between the multispecialty clinics and external physicians. This places special demands on effective communication.
- Complex, changing physician schedules include inpatient rounds, supervision of residents, and outreach clinic schedules.
- Participation in clinical trials complicates order entry, documentation, and billing.

For these reasons, the patient chart did not become irrelevant nearly as quickly in specialty practices as in our freestanding primary-care practices. Phased implementation meant that some practices were recording their notes in the EHR, while others were still using the paper chart. Despite this, we did not print notes from the EHR for inclusion in the paper chart. Rather, we notified clinicians that additional documentation was available in the EHR by way of a hand-stamped alert (placed by clerical personnel) on the appropriate page in the paper chart.

Ancillary Services

Ancillary testing and treatment areas located in many specialty practices also make these practices complex. For example, cardiology may operate a cardiac catheterization lab, EKG lab, and echo lab, along with a cardiac rehabilitation service. Neurology may operate an EEG lab and a sleep lab. Integrating these ancillary areas was often the most complex aspect of the implementation. Much of the complexity came from the fact that ancillary services may provide both inpatient and outpatient care. They often produce bills that include physician professional charges, technician fees, and equipment fees. They may perform studies using equipment and software that is unable to communicate electronically with the EHR.

To minimize these complexities, practice leaders choose the level of EHR function that ancillary areas will be allowed to use (e.g., results reviewing, messaging, order entry, documentation). The implementation team performs an analysis of the practice, makes recommendations, and implements decisions. For example, analysis of Cardiology's ancillaries revealed that there was no need for them to use any EHR function except messaging. Because of the clinical importance of EKG and echo lab results, that equipment was interfaced to the EHR. In the Ear, Nose and Throat practice audiology and speech-lab personnel need to use every EHR function, including limited order entry (for billing purposes).

Outreach Clinics

Many of our specialists see patients in outreach clinics located in primary-care practice sites, where the EHR was in use before the specialist's "home" practice had gone live. Since the workflows and configurations needed to support their use of the EHR were not yet implemented in their practice, they were not permitted to enter orders and document in the EHR in their outreach clinics. These outreach clinics needed to be included in the implementation planning of the specialty practices, to ensure that the system build reflected the workflows of both the home clinic and the outreach clinic and that shadowing support was available at the right times in both locations. Two weeks after go-live at their home practice site, specialists went live in their outreach clinics.

Special Purpose Software

Specialty practices often use one or more special-purpose clinical information systems to manage diagnostic equipment (ultrasound, EKG) or treatments (x-ray therapy, chemotherapy) or to handle the data needed for regulatory and clinical trials reporting. These systems are an important part of the practice's workflows and should be included in workflow analysis and redesign. (See Chapter 17.) The optimal approach to special-purpose software can range from including its function in the EHR to linking it to the EHR with an electronic interface to continuing to use it as a freestanding software application. In many cases, it is most cost-effective to continue to produce paper reports from the special-purpose system and allow clinicians to enter the results into the EHR (e.g., by entering "EEG wnl 5/04" in the patient summary) with or without scanning the report into the EHR. Table 16.1 provides examples of various solutions we have used.

Flexibility

Physicians who provide a mix of inpatient, outpatient, and outreach care have little time for EHR development and training. To make best use of their limited time, implementation teams met with physicians as early as 6:00 a.m. and as late as 9:00 PM (and on weekends).

Preparation

Even more than most adult learners, these physicians expect efficient, relevant analysis and training sessions. Training must focus on workflows and efficiency tools (e.g., note templates and order sets) developed specifically for their practice. (See Chapter 8.)

TABLE 16.1. Various Dispositions of Special-Purpose Software.

Specialty	Equipment/Auto mated System	Solution	Workflow
Cardiology	EKG	Interface	Phase 1: Link to text result. Print paper waveforms. Phase 2: Display waveforms in EHR. Discontinue printing.
Ophthalmology	Visual fields and topography	No interface	Since colors guide treatment decisions (and cannot be scanned), print results and file them in the paper record.
Dentistry	Dental X-rays	No interface	File films in paper chart.
Eyewear Center	Eyeglass ordering	Replaced by EHR.	EHR-based documentation.
MOHS Surgery	Home-grown database	FTP	Transfer key data elements into the EHR by FTP.
Endoscopy	Procedure documentation	Interface	(Scan documents into the EHR during interface development.)
Pulmonary, Sleep Lab, Neurophysiology	Various	Replaced by EHR.	Enter results entry directly into the EHR. The ordering physician receives the result in his in-basket.

Workflow Analysis

Implementation analysts spend 20 to 30 days in each practice, studying patients' movement from appointment scheduling through the visit to final checkout. Checklists of analytic questions (Appendix 11) improve efficiency and completeness, but do not replace sustained observation. For example, a nurse may report that, following check-in, a patient has been "roomed"—placed in the exam room to await the physician. This rooming process can be very practice-specific. In a urology clinic, a complete urinalysis may be performed routinely before a patient is placed in the exam room. In orthopedics, x-rays may be performed. To be effective, workflow design and user training must incorporate this level of detail. If these differences are not recognized until go-live, chaos can result.

Training

To avoid productivity losses, practice leaders mandated that no training sessions for specialty practices were to be scheduled for longer than two hours. This necessitated increased shadow training.

Special Implementation Challenges

Multispecialty Clinics

One frequent challenge is the multispecialty clinic in which two or more providers from different specialties provide care during a single patient encounter. For example, a patient in the Cleft Palate Clinic might be treated by a dentist, an oral surgeon, a psychiatrist, and a throat surgeon—in one exam room, with one check-in and one checkout. Before the EHR, each practice used separate workspaces, workflows, scheduling systems, documentation forms, and billing forms. As a result of the re-designed EHR workflows, the multispecialty clinics now have integrated scheduling, patient notification, patient records, billing records, and test results distribution to all providers.

Creating an integrated, multispecialty clinic requires the following steps (which take approximately one year to complete):

• Analysts need to understand the existing workflows. This is often difficult, since the various contributing practices may understand the clinic's existing workflows differently.
• Payers needed to be convinced to accept a single referral for multi-provider visits.
• A single, consistent clinic location must be agreed upon by all participating practices.
• Integrated billing with a single patient co-pay must be developed.
• If possible, scheduling should incorporate a single appointment type for each multispecialty clinic—comprised of one referral type, one appointment confirmation, one check-in, one EHR patient encounter, and one checkout.

Research Patients

Clinical researchers identified the following needs:

• A patient must be identified as a research participant any time the patient's record is accessed.

- Registries must be in list of patients participating in each study.
- Appropriate EHR access should be provided for authorized clinical trial reviewers.
- The patient's study-related medical history should be readily identifiable.
- Study-related charges need to be identified at the time of ordering (to enable ancillary and billing personnel to work effectively).
- The patient's providers must be kept unaware of the patient's assignment to the treatment or control group, particularly when they enter orders.

Clinical trial participant status is entered into patient demographics and is visible when front desk personnel take a patient message, schedule an appointment, or check a patient in. In addition, trial participation is documented on the patient's problem list with a unique diagnosis code. The comment field provides brief information about the trial, along with the research coordinator's contact information. Signed consent forms are scanned into the EHR and displayed with other consent forms. Trial documentation requirements are incorporated into note templates, which produce structured, searchable data. Authorized trial reviewers receive read-only access to the records of participants on the trial list. Their workflows and a customized security access agreement are incorporated into our Standard Operating Procedure. All of the identifiers are inactivated at the completion of the study (or the patient's withdrawal from it).

Billing for trial-related services proved to be the most complex task. Trial participants often have clinic visits that produce bills payable by their personal insurance, while other charges are solely for trial purposes and must be paid through trial funding. For example, a rheumatology patient could receive routine care for unrelated knee pain and then have blood samples drawn as part of a rheumatoid arthritis study. Ancillary systems (such as the lab) need prior notification to process the bills properly. The EHR generates electronic requisitions that display the necessary processing and billing information, which is also incorporated into billing documents.

Finally, trial medicines require management. We create a unique code for each trial drug or other orderable (e.g., "OKT47 trial"), since trial drugs rarely have a National Drug Code. In a blinded trial, the code only indicates that the patient received either the trial drug (or device) or the placebo. The study name, medicines (or devices) potentially received by the patient, and dispensing instructions, are listed on the patient's drug list. The EHR is configured to prevent the printing of a prescription for a trial drug or device, since all trial drugs (and placebos) are provided to patients according to the trial protocol.

Case Studies

Problem Escalation

Our Obstetrics & Gynecology Department incorporates several inpatient and outpatient practices, including maternal/fetal health and outreach clinics serving several counties with testing services (mammography, ultrasound, and andrology laboratory). When implementation analysts identified unexpectedly complex, interrelated workflows, they (along with the department's leaders) concluded that the original project timeline was unrealistically short. Using the issue escalation procedure, they recommended an extension of the timeline. The extension was approved by the CMIO, allowing the implementation team to develop a customized system build, with note templates and order sets designed for each sub-specialty.

Special-Purpose Software

Hematology/Oncology is another example of a complex, integrated practice with workflows that include outpatient clinics, a chemotherapy treatment unit, on-site laboratory and pharmacy, radiation therapy, palliative care, and inpatient practice. When Hematology/Oncology leaders questioned whether or not the EHR could adequately support these complexities, we conducted a formal needs assessment. Our conclusion was that the EHR would not adequately support the chemotherapy treatment unit for another three years. (See Chapter 2.) Following the planning process described in Chapter 17, the Hematology/Oncology practice developed a business plan to install chemotherapy management software optimized for managing hundreds of cancer treatment protocols.

Summary

Specialty practices differ from primary care in their team approach to patient care. That care may include multispecialty clinics and on-site ancillary departments, more complex physician schedules (due to inpatient rounding and outreach clinics), and the frequent need for special purpose software. Standardized implementation processes can take these differences into account and produce customized specialty implementations.

17
Special-Purpose Software

James M. Walker and Michael J. Komar

The rationale for special-purpose software to supplement the core EHR is compelling: There are many critical clinical processes that no general EHR software is (or soon will be) able to support effectively. (One example is integrated sub-systems for simultaneously documenting and coding procedures while capturing and labelling the associated images.) Unfortunately, most special-purpose software ends up costing an organization far more than is ever realized in benefits—financial or clinical. This chapter discusses methods for integrating special-purpose software with your core EHR in ways that will increase your odds of completing successful individual projects and of constructing an integrated, cost-effective EHR.

The Setting

Requests for special-purpose software almost invariably arise out of user dissatisfaction with the existing EHR. Frequently this dissatisfaction is the result of a "plain vanilla" implementation of the EHR that does not take adequate account of the workflows and information needs of specific user groups. Dissatisfaction may also stem from user ignorance of the functions available in the organization's currently implemented EHR. So requests for special-purpose software offer your team an opportunity to check the adequacy of your implementation and your training efforts—and to refine them both.

Another frequent cause of dissatisfaction with the EHR is the fact that many clinical information management needs go beyond the current (and sometimes developmental) scope of the EHR. This is an area where an effective partnership with your EHR vendor is critical. You need them to be organized enough to know what functions they plan to deliver and when—and honest enough to tell you. And you need them to deliver on schedule. Having a clear sense of whether and when new functions will be available is critical to making the business case for special-purpose software. If the new function will be available in six months, special-purpose software could not be selected and implemented in a shorter time frame. If the vendor has no plans to develop the function, it is a simple matter of estimating benefits and costs.

Another source of dissatisfaction arises out of EHRs' remarkable effectiveness at what they do well. Because of their high performance, users (as well as informaticians) may have trouble distinguishing between what is feasible (given inevitable resource constraints and organizational priorities), what is possible (in the absence of constraints), and what can as yet only be imagined.

Finally, special-purpose software may appear to be a better bargain than it is because many of the costs of a successful implementation are hidden from the customers. It is a rare sales presentation that includes any mention of the need for (or cost of) such critical project components as the needs assessment, process re-design, building and maintaining multiple electronic interfaces to other information systems, and planning for data security and confidentiality. Educating your internal customers regarding these considerations is a difficult, but critical, element of managing special-purpose software effectively. A written policy ratified and consistently enforced by senior clinical and operational leadership is a critical first step in the educational process. (See Appendix 12 for an example.)

Avoiding Chaos

It should be no surprise that special-purpose software strikes many clinicians and even some managers as a panacea. As opposed to the usual compromises among different stakeholders and the wait for implementation (or enhancement) of the core EHR, special-purpose software promises a rapid, focused solution to the needs of a specific set of users. But, while this narrow focus is the reason that special-purpose software exists, it has the potential to create chaos. This is because connectivity is critical to information system effectiveness. In the same way that a personally optimized telephone would be useless if it did not connect to the standard telephone system, special-purpose software—however perfectly designed for its users—must connect seamlessly to other information systems (e.g., EHR, laboratory, image management, scheduling, registration) to be usable. This is the main reason that most special-purpose software does not end up being used—even by the individuals who select it.

Understandably, connectivity seems relatively unimportant to users who request special-purpose software. They feel their own immediate needs vividly. They are unlikely to understand the importance of connectivity until, for example, multiple databases make creating a report difficult and expensive. In fact, it is often *their* customers (particularly other clinicians) who find the lack of connectivity between the special-purpose software and the core EHR unacceptable. For example, they may be mystified and impatient when echocardiography reports are not available in the EHR.

Lack of connectivity has multiple implications. The first is fragmentation of the EHR. For example, if colonoscopy results are not transmitted to the EHR, clinical-decision support to remind clinicians of a patient's need for colon cancer screening will be unworkable. Producing reports on the organization's performance on colon cancer screening will require accessing multiple databases, increasing the cost (or decreasing the quality and number) of reports that can be produced.

An obvious way to increase connectivity is to build electronic interfaces among information systems. Unfortunately, interfaces are unpredictably difficult and expensive to build and to maintain. As Clem McDonald, a leading EHR designer, implementer, and researcher observes, "These many different and cubby-holed systems present an enormous entropy barrier to the joining of patient data from many source systems in a single EHR. The work required in overcoming this entropy by interfacing to the many different islands and regularizing the data they contain has been more than most can afford. Medical data does not generate spontaneously within the medical record. It all comes from sources elsewhere in the world, and all of the obstacles and most of the work of creating an EHR relate to these external data sources and the transfer of their data into the EHR."[1]

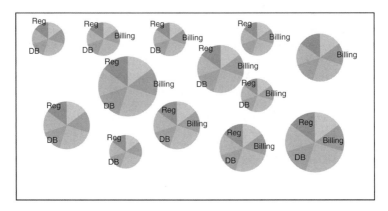

FIGURE 17.1. Multiple information systems with large numbers of redundant functions within a disorganized healthcare environment. The box represents the healthcare system, while each disc representing a self-contained information system with its own discreet functions: scheduling, laboratory, radiology etc. (DB = database, Reg = registration)

Figure 17.1 illustrates the way that non-interfaced, multiple clinical information systems require repeated performance of the same task, for example, entry of the patient registration.

Another hidden cost of special-purpose software is associated with "bullet-proofing" the system. Reducing downtime to an acceptable minimum, creating and testing a disaster recovery plan, and providing adequate information security are expensive of money and human resources. External regulations are not negotiable, but CDOs often make an implicit decision to operate such systems without effective fault tolerance and disaster recovery plans—a fact that users are typically unaware of until disaster strikes.

Special-Purpose Software and Confidential Address

You have invested substantial resources to assure that your core registration system protects patient confidentiality. One element of this protection is a place to record a patient's confidential address. However, a special-purpose application may not contain a confidential address field, exposing the organization to liability for failure to comply with the patients' request that you use their confidential address. Users of applications without interfaces from one of your core registration systems must consider the following questions:

Is the application ever used to register patients?

Is the patient ever contacted directly (by mail or phone) using the address or phone number stored in the application?

If yes, how will you accommodate patient requests that you use a confidential address or phone number?

Finally, implementing special-purpose software may delay the implementation and post-implementation optimization of the core EHR by draining away scarce human and financial resources from the core project. (Alternatively, it may give the organization one of the small wins that sustains the larger project.) More subtly, widespread use of special-purpose software can persuade the organization that specialized software and electronic interfaces are adequate substitutes for the organizational negotiation and process standardization that improved care quality and efficiency usually require.

Integrating Special-Purpose Software

Despite the risks that special-purpose-software systems carry with them, the answer is not to eliminate them, but rather to create a portfolio of software that meets your organization's needs.

The first step is to base your core EHR implementation on an organizationally agreed, prioritized list of clinical business needs. As you work down this priority list, your team will likely identify high priority needs that your core EHR vendor does not plan to support, at least not soon enough to meet your needs. Working this way, you will spend your implementation resources on the most strategic opportunities, whether core or special-purpose.

Of course, however closely you adhere to this principle, parts of your organization will undoubtedly follow the usual method of selecting special-purpose software: A physician will see a software demonstration at a national meeting and decide that it is the solution to a pressing need.

The problems with this method are many:

- The software may not do what the demonstration promised or implied it would.
- The software may be difficult to link to the core EHR.
- Even if the software works as promised, it may require extensive re-design of current workflows, with resulting organizational redesign costs.
- Since the demo didn't start with the organization's needs, it is unlikely that the organization's needs will be met—even by a "successful" project. (Or as Yogi Berra said, "If you don't know where you're going, you're likely to end up somewhere else.")
- Other users (e.g., pediatric cardiologists) will request a different, but essentially similar, software system because this one (e.g., chosen by adult cardiologists) does not meet their needs.
- The costs of the project will exceed expectations.
- Multiple electronic interfaces will be required. At least one will involve months of trying to get two prominent vendors to cooperate with your technical team.

Best Practice

Whether the EHR project team identifies a strategic need that will be unmet by the core EHR or a special-purpose software system is proposed by a user, the same process will increase the odds of the project producing measurable benefit to the organization.

- *Needs Assessment*—The first step is to document the needs that the special-purpose software will address. (See Chapter 2.) In the case of special-purpose software, it is particularly important to balance the needs of the practice (typically for increased local quality, efficiency, and profitability) with the organization as a whole (typically for improved service to internal and external customers and net financial benefit to the organization). It is also vital to ensure that all potential stakeholders have been consulted regarding their needs (e.g., pediatric and adult subspecialties, or multiple practices).

- *Executive Confirmation*—Executive leadership determines where the needs fit on IT's priority list. They also confirm that all relevant stakeholders have been included in the needs analysis.
- *Gap Analysis*—Identify the needs that cannot currently be met by the core EHR (and related software) and estimate when the needs will be met.
- *Market Assessment*—Assess special-purpose software products for their ability to meet the documented needs. Assess potential vendors for financial viability, for their likely longevity in the market, for their technical capability, and for their commitment to quality and customer service. We use well-known healthcare IT consultants to assess market viability, but since most of the vendors in question are small, new, and privately held, we have rarely gotten information that aided our final decision. For the market analysis, our most effective tool is a telephone conference call with current customers, supplemented by selective site visits. Vendors provide us with a list of ten organizations that are willing to be interviewed, and we conduct one-hour teleconferences with the three of them whose organizational needs seem most likely to be similar to ours. The conference calls are most effective if both sides include clinical, managerial, and technical participants. In our experience, three calls are enough to provide consistent and reliable information. (See Appendix 13 for an example of a reference call protocol.)
- *Information Security and Confidentiality*—Our information security and confidentiality office assesses the special-purpose software's compliance with regulations and industry best practices and estimates any costs of meeting internal and external standards.
- *Cost Estimates*—IT estimates the costs of purchasing, implementing, and maintaining the software system, as well as the likely impact on already prioritized IT projects.
- *Business Plan*—The requesting practice or department completes a business plan for the project, including a standard return-on-investment (ROI) projection and capital request.

Case Study—GI Endoscopy Documentation and Billing

Geisinger's Gastroenterology (GI) Department identified a report and image management system (provided by ProVation®) based upon the following identified needs:

- Minimize physician documentation time with a combination of optimized documentation and comprehensive, standardized clinical content.
- Bill accurately by way of:
  - payer-compliant documentation and
  - automated determination of billing codes.
- Acquire and store digital images efficiently.
- Add images to procedure reports to increase referring physician satisfaction.
- Capture and report standardized data for quality-improvement analysis, custom inquiries, and procedure performance logs for staff and trainees.
- Produce patient-education materials automatically.

Needs Assessment—As the clinical and operations leaders and IT analyst performed the needs assessment, they studied nurse and technician staffing, room turnover requirements, current patient flow, and available space for holding and recovery. They concluded that decreasing the time required for physician documentation would not increase patient throughput unless the endoscopy rooms could be cleaned and prepared for the next patient faster. To address this, the practice manager increased staffing and changed workflows to remove bottlenecks.

Executive Confirmation—Senior clinical and operations leaders met to review the needs and confirm that they represented a high priority for the organization.

Gap Analysis—Review of our EHR implementation plan and consultation with our EHR vendor confirmed that our core EHR would not contain this set of features for at least three years. We also confirmed that our PACS and imaging-archiving system (IDX-Stentor®) did not plan to provide this set of features.

Market Assessment—We were unable to find serious competitors in this market or any definite information regarding the vendor's financial viability. We were impressed with the results of the telephone conference calls, the performance of the software in real-world scenarios, the vendor's commitment to research and development, and their business plan for a set of products representing the full range of image-related procedures. (The latter is significant to us, because it offers the possibility of an integrated suite of applications with a single set of interfaces into and out of our interface engine. (See Figure 1.1, Chapter 11.)

Cost Estimates—Our IT analysts and the vendor collaborated on a set of technology-related costs for inclusion in the business plan.

Business Plan—Operational leaders projected the ROI conservatively, on the assumptions that: 1) there would be no interface for transmitting endoscopy results to the core EHR until after the project had succeeded, and 2) the system would be replaced by the core EHR in three years.

Results to-date include:

- Endoscopy room turnover time decreased from 15 minutes to five minutes.
- Procedure volume increased from 6,030 to 8,088 annually with no increase in rooms. (We did add one physician, who accounted for approximately 950 of the 2,058 added cases.)
- Net financial benefit of $265,000 for the first year.
- Physician documentation time decreased from 12 to two minutes per procedure.
- The electronic interface of procedure results to the EHR was completed without complications.

Since the GI endoscopy project, we have applied the policy to five other requests. One resulted in fuller use of the core EHR; two resulted in purchase of special-purpose software; and two have needs analyses underway. Clinical and administrative leaders are coming to regard the process as the appropriate way to do business.

Conclusion

The following practices will result in a proactive, high-performance approach to special-purpose software:

a. Identify and prioritize high-impact areas for special-purpose software.
b. Work a process like that outlined above, holding leaders responsible for business-plan results.

c. If possible, conduct pilot projects before committing the organization to interface costs.
d. Identify vendors with the culture, current products, and business plan that make them potential long-term partners. (See Chapter 13.) Focusing on a few such vendors will enable you to simplify business relationships and minimize interface costs.
e. Persuade your core EHR vendor to cooperate with the special-purpose software vendor.
f. Pool your experiences of special-purpose software and vendors with other organizations who use your core EHR. Your collective experiences, particularly with issues such as interfaces, will be mutually instructive.

Reference

1. McDonald C. The barriers to electronic medical record systems and how to overcome them. *J Am Med Informatics* 1997;4:213.

18
Optimizing Inpatient Care

Roy A. Gill and James M. Walker

Multiple efficacy studies suggest that hospital EHRs, and particularly physician order entry (CPOE), have significant potential to improve patient safety, care quality, and care process efficiency (1–5). Although real-world effectiveness studies confirming this are hard to find, there is widespread consensus among healthcare informaticians, payers, and health policy experts that inpatient EHRs are essential to quality healthcare. Unfortunately, inpatient EHRs continue to be difficult to implement (6–8), in large part because of the number and complexity of inpatient orders (9).

EHR Goals

The first step in developing an inpatient implementation plan is to agree on the 8 to 10 primary goals of the project. This will require the active participation of multiple stakeholders, including particularly hospital administration, physicians, nurses, admissions, pharmacy, and billing. In addition to guiding project development, the goals will determine the measures by which you evaluate the project's success and plan successive refinements. Each of the topics in this chapter is accompanied by representative goals, measures, and standards.

Standards of performance for EHRs and their users will become more stringent over the next several years, driven in part by the requirements of payers and regulators. More demanding performance standards will also be needed to support CDOs' ongoing development of safer, higher-quality care processes. Unless stated otherwise, the performance standards we present are for the first six months after go-live.

Implementation Plan

Based on our earlier experience with the "Big-Bang" and phased outpatient implementations, we planned a phased inpatient implementation. The acuity of inpatient problems and the complexity of inpatient care teams make it critical that any negative impact on workflow efficiency be minimal and brief, so a phased implementation is particularly attractive in this setting.

Because our outpatient EHR includes test results (lab and radiology, inpatient and outpatient) as well as outpatient histories, notes, orders, and radiology results (inpatient and outpatient), the effective first phase of the inpatient EHR project was the use of the outpatient EHR to access inpatient test results. Some providers even used the outpatient EHR to create inpatient admission histories and physical examinations, which they printed and placed in the inpatient (paper) chart.

A second peculiarity of our situation is that our physicians (and outpatient-clinic support staff) became familiar with the EHR before the hospital's nurses, who had previously used the EHR minimally to access laboratory results and not at all for messaging.

Based on all these considerations, we divided the implementation into three formal phases: facilitated information review, provider order entry and documentation, and nursing documentation and medication administration.

Phase One: Facilitated Information Review

The first formal phase of the implementation was the presentation of clinical information organized into patient lists. This allows clinicians to review the status of their patients in a single overview. Status icons indicate the presence of unreviewed and abnormal results and un-reviewed notes with links to the full text. Lists are created automatically according to hospital unit, service, practice group, and by the attending physician to whom the patient is linked in the ADT (inpatient registration) system. Users are also able to create custom lists (e.g., to facilitate monitoring of discharged patients, particularly patients with tests pending on discharge).

Because the patient lists are fed by the hospital's ADT system, analysis began in the admissions department. First, the implementation team reviewed the information created by the ADT system (e.g., patient census by hospital unit) and how that information could be presented to EHR users. Next, the team interviewed all types of clinicians and attended patient rounds to identify information needs and to assess the tools that were in use to track patient location. Finally, they reviewed the EHR software to determine the options available for patient list organization and display of information. For example, Table 18.1 shows the header that organizes the patient list view.

Based on clinician feedback, we positioned the "New Result" and "New Note" columns that display dynamic, clinically significant information, to the center of the display for maximum visibility. Columns containing information needed to identify the patients and their physician(s) were moved to the left, where the Western eye begins scanning. Columns containing less critical, less dynamic information were moved to the right.

The second major part of phase one was presentation of test results for review. Here, the primary task was organizing the various lab results into clinically meaningful groupings, such as Diabetes, Cardiology, and Infectious Disease (see Table 18.2). In addition, we placed some of the most commonly ordered test panels (such as general chemistry and CBC) at the top of the display, for easy access. (See Chapter 7.)

Phase Two: Provider Order Entry and Documentation

Based on our experience with outpatient phased implementation—where physicians requested the merging of order entry and documentation into a single phase—and repeated provider requests for rapid implementation of both order entry and

TABLE 18.1. Patient List Layout.

Room/ Bed	Patient Name	Service	Attending Physician	New Result	New Note	Medical Record #	Age	Gender	Adm Date	Adm Time	Patient Type

TABLE 18.2. Cardiology Lab Test Results.

Troponin T
Troponin I
CK
MB fraction
Chol
HDL
LDL
Triglycerides
Hours fasting
Lipid Phenotype
Apo A
Apo B
ApoB/ApoA Ratio
CRP (hs)
Homocysteine
Pro BNP

documentation, we plan to implement provider order entry and documentation together.

Documentation

To minimize the confusion that would result if some documents were available in the paper chart and others in the EHR (particularly if this varied from unit to unit or service to service), we began the implementation with note types that are only infrequently available in the paper chart during the patient's hospital stay—operative notes and ED discharge summaries. (See box.) This allowed the implementation team and clinicians to resolve most implementation issues (including user training) before an accelerated extension of the rollout to implementation of daily notes documentation (which comprises the bulk of a paper chart). Since clinicians are already accustomed to using the EHR to access results (including pathology and documents), we do not print electronic notes for inclusion in the paper chart.

Physician Documentation Pilot

An ideal inpatient documentation pilot project would have:

- A capable, motivated leader.
- Controlled scope.
  - Require minimal workflow alterations for related users and systems.
  - Involve a small group of users.
  - Be geographically well defined.
  - Involve a single document type.
- High clinical value.

- Achieve significant financial benefit.
- Address an outpatient need simultaneously.

Using the EHR to document operative (and procedure) notes before the surgeon leaves the operating suite met all these criteria for us. The project had minimal negative impact on providers. Users did not need to worry about using different flows in different areas of the hospital.

The implementation team made every effort to simplify the first phase of the project (leaving almost all related processes unchanged). Even so, the large number of connected processes required a detailed analysis of every workflow (patient movement, scheduling, paper flows) in the operative suite. It also required a detailed analysis of information exchange among referring physicians, surgeons, surgical practices, the Medical Record Department, and the Billing Department. This analysis helped define the goals of the project, which included:

- Availability of the operative note in the EHR within one hour of the completion of the procedure.
- Elimination of the need for a written interval operative note.
- Improved completeness of operative notes (as measured by the inclusion of patient identification, attestation of the surgeons, and supervision information).
- Real-time transmission of the operative note to the Billing Department for claim submission.
- Real-time transmission to the medical records department.

Results

Most of the work involved defining methods for creating and approving note templates, learning the general workflows in the operating suites (understanding how and where the op note was created, how patients are scheduled and how the schedule is used), and analyzing how the operative note would get to the paper chart and to referring providers.

Barriers

- The main barrier (and benefit) was the need for various groups who were not used to working together (i.e., surgeons, IT, billing, operating suite management and medical records staff) to cooperate on this project. Building this cooperation required daily communication, especially between the lead surgeon and the implementation team, for several weeks.
- A particularly difficult decision was whether or not to include ICD-9 and CPT-4 codes within the operative notes. The surgeons were confident that they could pick correct codes and thereby improve the quality of the information in their notes. The billing department was concerned that if the code chosen needed to be changed, it would require creating an addendum to the medical record, potentially complicating billing. Our compromise was to have the surgeon choose the diagnosis (written in the language of ICD-9 and CPT-4 but without the numerical code). For billing purposes, coders subsequently choose the code that most accurately represents the services rendered.

To assure complete notes, we began by having physicians and nurses, the medical-records staff, and the billing department validate the general outline of a master template. The Op Note template consists of the following sections:

- Patient
- Date
- Pre- and post-op diagnoses
- Operators
- Procedure performed
- Pertinent history
- Description of operation
- Attestation of which phases of the operation the staff physician participated in (performed procedure, performed part of the procedure, observed, etc.) This is needed where residents and other trainees have varying involvement in surgical cases.

Once the general outline was agreed upon, the same groups of stakeholders cooperated to develop templates for specific diagnoses and procedures (e.g., operative note for laparoscopic cholecystectomy), starting with high-volume procedures. The team identified appropriate content by reviewing patient charts and the templates that transcriptionists use to format dictated notes and by interviewing physicians. Then clinicians and staff from medical records, billing, and the legal department validated the final products.

Efficiency Tools

If they are to be effective, documentation tools—particularly order sets and note templates—must be easier and faster to use than writing or dictating. One way to accomplish this is to focus on the elements of the history, physical examination, and procedure that need to be documented because they will influence providers' decision making. The many clinical prediction rules (CPRs) that have been validated and published in the last decade provide one good place to start in the development of efficiency tools. (See Chapter 15 for Deyo's CPR for new-onset low-back pain.) The Ottawa ankle rule is an example that is particularly relevant to the emergency department (10–11).

Defaulting

Defaulting answers to their usual state (e.g., a normal lung exam in an elective surgical patient) is another important way to save user time. Since all possible selections cannot be anticipated, selection lists should routinely include "wildcards," that is, places to add free text. Researchers and administrators may fear a loss of structured data when this flexibility is available, but early research suggests that EHR users are unlikely to switch from a faster (templated) to a slower form of documentation (typing or even dictation) (12).

Goal: Rapid Documentation
Measures:
a. Time from procedure to availability of the note to other caregivers (Standard: 90% within one hour)
b. STAT Radiology Studies—Time from when the patient leaves the examination room to when the final report is available to the ordering physician (Standard:90% within 30 minutes)

c. *Time from order completion to order receipt in the pharmacy. (Standard: 90% reduction) (13)*

d. *Users will prefer EHR documentation tools to writing or dictation (Standard: 80%)*

Goal: Cost-savingMeasure: Lines of inpatient transcription. (Standards: 30% reduction at 6 months after go-live; 70% reduction at 12 months)

Ancillary Documentation

Other important patient-care activities (such as nutrition assessment, fall prevention, and documentation of advanced directives) are incompletely documented and are expensive to audit using paper charts. By including orders for these services in admission order sets, providing templates for documenting the services, and providing performance reports, the EHR can support improved performance.

Goal: Assess patient nutrition as appropriate.
Measures:
a. *Document assessment of patient's nutritional status (or contraindication) within 24 hours of admission. (Standard: 95%)*
b. *Document the nutritional status of intensive-care patients every 48 hours (Standard: 100%)*

Goal: Assess risk for falling and plan preventive measures as indicated.
Measures:
a. *Document fall-risk assessment (or contraindication) within 24 hours of admission. (Standard: 95%)*
b. *Document fall prevention plan (as indicated) within 24 hours of admission. (Standard: 95%)*

Goal: Give every competent patient the opportunity to choose advanced directives.
Measure: Document discussion and patient decision (or contraindication) within 24 hours of admission. (Standard: 100%)

Provider Communication

Goal: Communicate with referring and primary care providers in a timely manner.
Measure: Discharge Summaries are available to referring providers and primary care physicians within 24 hours of discharge. (Standard: 95% of summaries received by providers who use electronic communications (i.e., fax machines, or secure e-mail).

Document Distribution

In addition to streamlining the billing process, the EHR can make clinical documentation (e.g., operative notes) available for clinical use far more quickly than before. In the case of some note types (e.g., history and physicals, op notes) this can have the added virtue of making written interval notes unnecessary.

Goal: Decrease time to distribution of clinical documentation.
Measures:
a. *Operative notes (outpatient and inpatient) are completed and distributed within one hour of the end of the procedure. (Standard: 90%)*
b. *Specific note templates are available for surgical procedures. (Standard: 90% of procedures performed).*

Order Entry

Large numbers of usable order sets are frequently cited as the most important efficiency tool for inpatient EHRs (although we are aware of no studies) (14-16). Successful implementation teams typically recommend approximately 500 order sets to
support go-live. However, Payne, et al, reported that only 53% of their individual
"quick orders" (e.g., for standard doses of commonly used medicines) and order sets
were used. Although they were unable to capture data regarding which orders were
used by whom, they did observe that users in focused domains that require numerous
orders (e.g., PAs working in orthopedic surgery) are prone to be heavy users (17)).

The topics and contents of order sets are typically defined by clinicians, but other
departments may recognize the need for a particular order or component of a set as
well (e.g., billing, medical records, quality improvement). The pharmacy makes important contributions to the inpatient EHR, particularly in the case of complex orders,
such as total parenteral nutrition (TPN) orders. A typical order set has the following
components:

- Diagnosis (often with multiple choices available)
- Orders
  - Standard
  - Optional
- Link to note template
- Patient instructions

The implementation team identifies appropriate content for specific order sets by
reviewing paper order sets, the templates that transcriptionists use to format dictated
notes, and patient charts (to identify which paper order sets are actually used). They
also interview clinicians, particularly the Domain Experts who regularly build orders
sets for their outpatient practices. (See Chapter 9, Clinical Decision Support, for a
description of domain experts.) We solicit suggestions from organizational sources of
best practice recommendations, such as Pharmacy, Laboratory, Infection Control, Risk
Management, Utilization Management and Billing. Finally, we review published
sources, such as validated quality measures (18), clinical practice guidelines, and reports
of clinical trials.

A number of factors are important to remember about order sets:

1. *Speed is paramount.* If order sets don't speed the task of initiating orders, the implementation will be endangered (7, 19, 20).
2. *Simplicity contributes to speed.*
3. *Users need help finding order sets.* You will create hundreds of order sets. Users will
   use different strategies for finding them (as well as other EHR elements).
   a. Naming: Based on our experience and that of other organizations, most users find
      order sets by pattern matching, that is, by typing the first few letters of a name
      and letting the EHR find candidate choices. This makes the names and synonyms
      you give to order sets critical. (See Chapter 7.)
   b. Hierarchies: At least a significant minority of EHR users prefer to find EHR
      elements in ordered hierarchies (e.g., locating AAA Repair in the Vascular
      Surgery sub-section of the Surgery section). For these users, both usable names
      and consistent organization are important. Creating hierarchies that are optimal
      for all users is not possible. For this reason, your EHR software should allow the
      listing of any element in multiple places. For instance, Carpal Tunnel Release
      should be accessible in both the Orthopedics and Plastic Surgery sub-sections.

4. *Users come to order sets with multiple needs.*
   a. To initiate a care pathway (e.g., post-surgical orders)
   b. To order a single item (e.g., a head CT with or without contrast)
   c. To arrange specialty care (e.g., wound care)
   d. To clarify the details of an order (e.g., what options are available for TPN?)
5. *Order Sets require management after implementation.*
   a. *Content Review:* Although a rigorous CDS review process appears to be the exception rather than the rule (21), potentially out-of-date order sets (which at least appear to suggest interventions which are no longer standard-of-care) pose risks both to patients and to CDOs. The only study we are aware of concluded that 10% of guidelines were no longer "valid" 3.6 years after their promulgation. The authors recommended guideline review every three years (22). In view of the enormous number of CDS rules involved, (Regenstrief estimates that they have 64,000 in production (21)), content review will only be feasible when computer applications are available to monitor when rules need review and who is responsible to review them.
   b. *Functionality review:* As EHR software continues to become more usable, older order sets (and individual orders) will need to be reviewed to ensure that they are fully optimized. Tagging order sets in order to audit their use will enable the CDO to update tools in a rational order, beginning with the most frequently used. However, this approach will miss order sets that support a critical activity but are unused because they are unusable. To manage these, we keep a spreadsheet of needed clinical decision support tools that are currently not feasible or too difficult to use to be effective. (See the Content Matrix in the The Decision Support Implementers' Workbook (23).)

Order Management

Once entered, orders must be transmitted with appropriate urgency to nurses, other providers (e.g., consultants), and ancillary departments (such as laboratory and radiology). The exact status of the order should be readily available, saving the considerable time that clinicians currently spend locating information on the status of orders (24). While digital paging shows promise for speeding order reporting (25, 26), real-world use of such systems will depend on development by enterprise EHR vendors and expensive paging equipment upgrades to be effective (27).

Verbal Orders

Verbal orders are a potential source of error (although they may be safer than written orders (28)). Verbal orders also have the potential to short-circuit clinical decision support by removing physicians from exposure to the alerts and reminders triggered by an order. Using the EHR, physicians will be able to enter orders personally from almost any location (e.g., office, home, any computer connected to the Internet), decreasing the need for verbal orders. The EHR can also send verbal orders to the provider's inbasket for signature and automatically report to designated managers if orders are not signed within 24 hours.

Goal: Timely electronic authentication of verbal orders.
Measures:
a. *Proportion of non-emergency orders entered by providers (Standard: 100%).*
b. *Proportion of verbal orders finalized within 24 hours (Standard: 100%).*

Patient Education

Forster et al., found that 20% of patients discharged from a large teaching hospital suffered a care-related adverse event following discharge. Two-thirds of the adverse events could have been prevented or minimized by better communication. Hard-to-understand discharge summaries were identified as one of the main causes of failed communication (29).

The EHR will enable hospitals to provide patients with standardized discharge instructions that include potential adverse effects of care and contact information in lay language.

Goal: More useful patient instructions at discharge
Measures:
a. *Discharge instructions include potential adverse events associated with discharge medications which occur more frequently than with placebo (where this information is available). (Standard: 70% at go-live; 85% at 6 months post-go-live; 100% at one year)*
b. *Discharge instructions include potential adverse events associated with procedures. (Standard: 85% at go-live; 100% at 6 months)*
c. *Discharge instructions include instructions regarding whom to call if any adverse event is suspected. (Standard: 100% at go-live)*
d. *Discharge instructions are written at the 6th-grade reading level. (Standard: 85% at six months post-go-live; 100% at one year)*
e. *Patients find their discharge instructions helpful. (Standard: 90% of patients find them "helpful" or "very helpful," 4 or 5 on a five-point Likert scale.)*

Phase Three: Nursing Documentation

Documentation in an EHR has been shown to improve nurses' performance and job satisfaction in several studies (30–32). In particular, two recent studies have found that use of an EHR allowed nurses to decrease time spent on clerical work and to increase time spent on patient care. (33, 34) As the book went to press, we were beginning the analysis for inpatient nursing documentation, using the methods discussed in this and earlier chapters.

Evolving Clinician Feedback

Full involvement of physicians and other clinicians in every phase of an inpatient implementation is one of the universally agreed factors for success (14, 16, 35). At the beginning of our inpatient project (in 2002), this principle had been fully embodied at Geisinger for five years—through the leadership of the CMIO; the active support of the CEO, CMO, and other physician executives; physician membership on oversight, feedback, and clinical decision support committees; domain experts (generally physicians) charged with building note templates and order sets for individual practices; and two physician informaticians who spend 80% of their time each on informatics projects (primarily the EHR).

Pressure on physicians to increase their patient care activities and billings has been steadily increasing. In addition, the physicians who are most perceptive and organizationally aware in their assessments of the EHR are prone to become leaders in other domains, further limiting their availability for meetings. In 2003 (early in the inpatient implementation), these converging trends prompted us to create a virtual feedback group as an adjunct to our face-to-face multidisciplinary feedback team (which has two to six physicians in attendance at its meetings). The members agree to respond (within one week) to e-mailed questions that the face-to-face team or the CMIO believe need more wide-based physician input before decision. Ninety-five percent of the twenty physicians we invited were eager to support the EHR project in this way. Their feedback has consistently been timely, often enabling the project to move ahead more quickly and effectively than would otherwise have been the case.

Electronic Consent Calendar

EHR implementation projects raise literally thousands of questions that vary in complexity, controversy, and system implications. Some require careful research by multiple departments (Legal, Billing, Information Security and Information Confidentiality) and decision by executive forums. Others are so numerous and have such seemingly obvious answers that they must be decided using minimum resource. Deciding where a given question lies on this spectrum often requires considerable judgment.

One method we use for triaging questions is the electronic consent calendar. This is a list of proposals that the development team believes have significant benefits and negligible risks. The list is distributed by e-mail one week before the feedback group's scheduled meeting. If a recipient sees any potential problem with any of the proposals, he is encouraged to note that fact by return e-mail. The proposal is then removed from the consent calendar and put on the meeting's agenda for consideration. Consent calendar proposals that elicit no comment are implemented without further discussion. This method allows feedback groups to focus on issues that need their attention, at the same time reducing the risk that significant issues are being overlooked.

Supporting An Inpatient Go-Live

Go-live support for the inpatient EHR differs from outpatient in a number of ways. Most obviously, training and support must serve users working around the clock. To meet this need, we provide training on all three shifts. Second and third shift training is provided primarily by nurse educators trained by the EHR team. We provide on-site support 24 × 7 for two to five days past go-live (two days for Phase One and five days for the order entry and documentation implementation). Extra staff support the increased physician use of the EHR that occurs during pre-rounding and morning rounds. We provide a second-shift telephone trainer on call (See Chapter 12.) for two weeks after go-live.

Particularly in the inpatient setting, EHR users are dealing with urgent and emergent patient needs, often while they are sleep-deprived. Conflict resolution skills are particularly important for inpatient trainers. In addition, the CMIO and other leaders will occasionally need to remind some clinicians of the basics of professional behavior.

Summary

Implementing an effective inpatient EHR requires careful attention to the information needs of complex healthcare teams as they provide time-pressured care to acutely ill patients. Users will need hundreds of efficient order sets and note templates at go-live. Multiple administrative needs must be accommodated. Setting explicit, widely agreed-upon goals for the project will enable the leaders of various departments to work together toward implementation success and to identify opportunities for ongoing improvement.

References

1. Gardner R. CPOE. AMIA Fall Symposium. Los Angeles: AMIA; 2000.
2. Tierney W, Miller M, Overhage M. Physician inpatient order writing on microcomputer workstations. *JAMA* 1993;269:379–383.
3. Overhage J. A randomized trial of corollary orders to prevent errors of omission. *J Am Med Informatics* 1997;4:364.
4. Mekhjian H, Rajee R, Kumar P, Kuehn L. Immediate Benefits Realized Following Implementation of Physician Order Entry at an Academic Medical Center. *J Am Med Informatics* 2002;9:529–539.
5. Bates DW, Gawande AA. Improving Safety with Information Technology. *New Engl J Med* 2003;348:2526–2534.
6. Massaro T. Introducing physician order entry at a major academic medical center: I. Impact on organizational culture and behavior. *Academic Medicine* 1993;68:20–25.
7. Massaro T. Introducing physician order entry at a major academic medical center: II. Impact on medical education. *Academic Medicine* 1993;68:25–30.
8. Versel N. Cedars-Sinai goes back to paper orders. Modern Physician online; 2003. www.modernphysician.com/news.cms?newsId=433
9. Sittig D. Computer-based order entry: the state of the art. *J Am Med Informatics Assoc* 1994; 1:108.
10. Boutis K, LK, Jaramillo D. Sensitivity of a clinical examination to predict need for radiography in children with ankle injuries: a prospective study. *Lancet* 2001;358:2118–21.
11. Bachmann LM, Kolb E, Koller MT. Accuracy of Ottawa ankle rules to exclude fractures of the ankle and mid-foot: systematic review. *Br Med J* 2003;326:417.
12. Patel V. Interface Design for Health Care Environments: The Role of Cognitive Science. AMIA Fall Symposium. Orlando, FL: AMIA; 1998.
13. iHealthBeat. North Carolina hospital scores with CPOE, 2003. http://www.ihealthbeat.org/index.cfm?Action=dspItem&itemID=99060
14. Ahmad A, Teater P, Bentley TD. Key Attributes of a Successful Physician Order Entry System Implementation in a Multi-hospital Environment. *J Am Med Informatics* 2002;9:16–24.
15. Payne TH, Hoey PJ, Nichol P. Preparation and Use of Pre-Constructed Orders. *J Am Med Informatics* 2003;10:322–329.
16. Metzger J, Fortin J. CPOE in Community Hospitals. www.chcf.org:FCG; 2003.
17. Payne TH. Order Set Use. Personal Communication; 2003.
18. Wachter R, UCSF-Stanford University Evidence-based Practice Center. Making Health Care Safer: A Critical Analysis of Patient Safety Practices and Chapter 25. Beta-blockers and Reduction of Perioperative Cardiac Events. Rockville, MD: Agency for Healthcare Research and Quality, Contract No. 290–97–0013; 2001. Report No.: Evidence Report/Technology Assessment, No. 43.
19. Ornstein C. Hospital Heeds Doctors, Suspends Use of Software. Los Angeles: *Times*; January 22, 2003.
20. McDonald C. The Regenstrief Medical Record System: 30 years of learning. AMIA Annual Symposium. Washington, DC; 2001.

21. Overhage J, Sittig D. CDS rules management. Personal communication, 2003.
22. Shekelle P, Ortiz E, Rhodes S, Morton SC, Eccles MP, Grimshaw JM, et al. Validity of the Agency for Healthcare Research and Quality Clinical Practice Guidelines: How Quickly Do Guidelines Become Outdated? *JAMA*. 2001;286:1461–1467.
23. Content Matrix in The Decision Support Implementers' Workbook. www.himss.org/asp/cds_workbook.asp
24. McKnight LK, Stetson PD, Bakken S, Curran C, Cimino JJ. Perceived Information Needs and Communication Difficulties of Inpatient Physicians and Nurses. *J Am Med Informatics* 2002;9:S64-S69.
25. Tate KE, Gardner RM, Scherting K. Nurses, pagers, and patient-specific criteria: three keys to improved critical value reporting. *Proc Annu Symp Comput Appl Med Care* 1995:164–8.
26. Poon E, Kuperman G, Fiskio J. Real-Time Notification of Laboratory Data Requested by Users through Alpha-Numeric Pagers. AMIA Fall Symposium. Washington, D.C.; 2001.
27. McDonald C, Overhage J, Tierney W. The Regenstrief Medical Record System (RMRS): Physician use for input and output and Web browser-based computing.AMIA Fall Sumposium. Washington, D.C.; 1996.
28. Shojania KG, Duncan BW, McDonald KM, Wachter RM. Safe but Sound: Patient Safety Meets Evidence-Based Medicine. *JAMA* 2002; 288:508–13.
29. Forster AJ, Murff HJ, Peterson JF, Gandhi TK, Bates DW. The Incidence and Severity of Adverse Events Affecting Patients after Discharge from the Hospital. Ann Intern Med 2003; 138:161–167.
30. Case J, Mowry M, Welebob E. The Nursing Shortage—Can Technology Help? First Consulting Group; 2002.
31. Eurlings F, Asten A, Cozijn H. Effects of a nursing information system in 5 Dutch hospitals. *Stud Health Technol Inform* 1997;46:50–55.
32. Oniki TA, Terry P, Clemmer MD, Pryor TA. The Effect of Computer-generated Reminders on Charting Deficiencies in the ICU. *J Am Med Informatics* 2003;10:177–87.
33. iHealthBeat. Online system reduces nurse documentation time, 2002. http://www.ihealthbeat.org/index.cfm?Action=dspItem&itemID=98572
34. Wong DHP, MD; Gallegos, Yvonne RN, MSN; Weinger, Matthew B. Changes in intensive care unit nurse task activity after installation of a third-generation intensive care unit information system. *Critical Care Medicine* 2003;31:2488–2494.
35. Ash JS, Stavri PZ, Kuperman GJ. A Consensus Statement on Considerations for a Successful CPOE Implementation. *J Am Med Informatics* 2003;10:229–234.

Additional Reading

Ash JS, Stavri PZ, et al. (2003). "A Consensus Statement on Considerations for a Successful CPOE Implementation." JAMIA 10:229–234 (2003).
A carefully derived set of best practices primarily relevant to inpatient implementations.
Metzger J, Fortin J (2003). CPOE in Community Hospitals, CHCF FCG.
A compilation of best practices based on case studies.
Case J, Mowry M, et al. (2002). The Nursing Shortage—Can Technology Help?, First Consulting Group.
Provides a useful overview of EHR functions (and other technologies) that improve nursing workflows.

19
Extending EHR Access to Patients

KIMBERLY A. ROKITA, JOAN E. TOPPER, MICHAEL C. LAMPMAN, and DAVID L. YOUNG

Why Extend Access?

"A former Fox News television producer sued one of the nation's largest pharmaceutical firms claiming the hepatitis A vaccine he received failed to protect him from the debilitating liver disease. Fox News hired veteran journalist Claude Novak and assigned him to cover the war in Afghanistan in 2001. Novak received travel vaccinations at a[n] Executive Health Exams International clinic in New York. Merck & Co produced the hepatitis A vaccine Novak received. Novak became seriously ill while working in Pakistan from November 2001 until January 2002. When he got home, Novak received belated notification the Merck hepatitis A vaccine had been recalled because it was ineffective and would not protect him against the disease. Medical tests later determined Novak had contracted hepatitis A and had suffered severe liver damage. Novak continues to suffer symptoms of the disease and has been unable to work." (1).

A practice with CPOE and secure e-messaging can run a database search to identify patients who received an ineffective lot of the vaccine and send patients a message that is readable anywhere there is Internet access. At the time of the Hepatitis A vaccine recall (2001), only half of our outpatient practices were using CPOE and none had secure e-messaging. We ran a search of the patients in the EHR-enabled clinics and notified them by U.S. mail and telephone.

Giving patients electronic access to their EHR and secure E-messaging via a patient EHR has the potential to revolutionize healthcare. With easier access to more information, patients can participate more effectively in their care. (Mr. Novak could have been notified in Pakistan that he needed another shot.) Both patients and practices can create more efficient ways of working together (for example, with prescription renewals requested by the patient one evening and processed by the patient's practice the next morning). These information services can support healthcare of a quality and efficiency that is not possible without it. This chapter will provide pointers on how to begin.

A Note on Terminology

The application we use, MyChart®, is a secure, Web-based application that allows patients to view portions of their electronic medical record and to exchange secure e-messages with their physician's practice. It is provided by Epic Corporation® as a part of their EHR application suite. We will use the phrase "patient EHR" to refer to this service of providing patients access to their EHR and secure e-messaging.

Goals

Our e-health strategy is to use the Internet and the EHR to provide new healthcare services that will delight our patients, improve their healthcare, create workflow efficiencies, and give us a competitive advantage in our market area. Our patient-related goals for the patient EHR—based on the Institute of Medicine's report, "Crossing the Quality Chasm" (2)—are threefold: (1) to provide patients access to central elements of their EHR, (2) to provide a comprehensive library of self-care information, and (3) to offer an efficient, secure and accountable way for patients to communicate with Geisinger practices.

Patient Preferences

Access to the Internet is increasing—at work, in public places, and at home. For increasing numbers of people, e-messaging is a preferred communication channel. Particularly significantly for healthcare, the fastest growing group of Internet users is women over the age of 65 (3).

Patient surveys, literature searches and reviews of existing patient EHRs helped us to determine the content and features that would be most useful to our patients.

A survey conducted in our outpatient practices in 2000, found the following preferences (Figure 19.1):

Prefer to use a patient EHR for

Asking health questions	77%
Managing appointments	71%
Requesting prescription renewals	71%
Accessing test results	70%

A National Harris Interactive poll published in 2002 reflected similar preferences (4).

Contents

We provide the following elements of the EHR to patients:

- Healthcare histories (including the active problem list)
- Immunizations (in printable form)
- Allergies

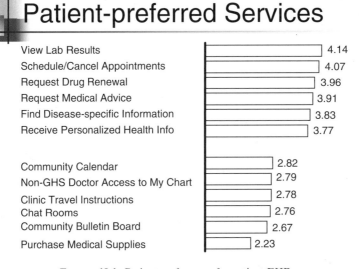

Patient-preferred Services

View Lab Results	4.14
Schedule/Cancel Appointments	4.07
Request Drug Renewal	3.96
Request Medical Advice	3.91
Find Disease-specific Information	3.83
Receive Personalized Health Info	3.77
Community Calendar	2.82
Non-GHS Doctor Access to My Chart	2.79
Clinic Travel Instructions	2.78
Chat Rooms	2.76
Community Bulletin Board	2.67
Purchase Medical Supplies	2.23

FIGURE 19.1. Patient preferences for patient EHR.

- Medicines with dosages and explanations of uses and potential adverse effects
- Lab test results with interpretations
- Appointments, with instructions (e.g., "Bring all medicines you are taking")
- Health reminders (e.g., "LDL check due." with the due date)
- Links to other high-quality sources of patient information (such as Medline Plus)
- A place for the patient to keep private notes

From Jargon to Patient Understanding

Any provision of personal healthcare information to patients (whether face-to-face or electronic) must be preceded by a thoughtful assessment of how the information and its method of delivery are likely to affect the patient. For example, seeing an abnormal laboratory result (however clinically benign) could be frightening to a patient if the results are viewed in the EHR prior to the provider's interpretation. For this reason, the patient EHR will not release results to the patient before the ordering provider releases them.

We currently display the 32 most frequently ordered laboratory tests. These 32 represent approximately 90% of all test orders. Our physician informaticians write explanations of each test, with the goal of making the descriptions readable (at the sixth-grade reading level) and clinically informative, while avoiding language that suggests alarming (and unlikely) possible reasons for an abnormal result. The descriptions are also edited by lay people for readability. Patient feedback groups and online survey questionnaires indicate that patients value access to test results, sometimes find the results worrisome, but want access to even more results (unpublished). We have also translated 1,500 ICD-9 diagnosis codes (which were designed for billing and are often difficult even for physicians to interpret) into natural English (e.g., "high blood pressure" instead of "benign hypertension").

Because they are (necessarily) jargon-filled and often preliminary in their content, we do not display clinical notes, such as office visit notes. Radiology reports also have great potential to create misunderstanding. Summary documents, such as letters and discharge summaries, are more likely to be useful to patients, but are still not available to our patients since we cannot yet separate them from other types of notes.

General Content

Non-clinical content provides additional value for patients:

- Practice hours of operation
- Travel directions
- General interest healthcare news stories
- Community healthcare events (e.g., Breast Cancer Awareness Month)

Messaging

To preserve the safety features of existing message-management workflows (that is, if the patient's primary physician is out, the message is routed to another provider) and decrease training needs, our e-messaging workflows reflect prior workflows. Analysts observed how phone calls were handled in a practice and arranged for e-messages to be routed in the same ways.

Typically, phone calls do not go directly to a provider. They are usually triaged by front office or nursing personnel, depending on the type of call—administrative (scheduling a visit) or clinical (requesting a prescription renewal). Since messages go to pools, they do not go unanswered when an individual clerk, nurse, or provider is unavailable.

When patients send messages they are reminded of the following guidelines:

- Do not include sensitive health information you do not want office support staff to read.
- Do not use e-messaging for urgent matters.
- The e-message is likely to become part of your electronic medical record.
- Normal turnaround time is one business day.

Implementation

With the outpatient EHR in full use and an understanding of patient needs, we turned to implementing the patient EHR. The implementation team developed procedures for giving patients access to the system and for responding to their e-messages. We began with primary-care practices to simplify the routing of patient messages if the patient has more than one Geisinger doctor. We deferred pediatric access until a later phase of the project because of the legal and social complexities of providing EHR access to children. (Some organizations have concluded that the complexities—which vary from state to state—preclude providing pediatric access.) We also deferred large-scale marketing until we had preliminary information on the effects of the patient EHR on physician and support staff workloads. We also needed time to streamline technical support processes, particularly online patient registration. We did provide marketing materials (including posters, pamphlets, a specially designed screen saver for computers in exam rooms, and a recorded telephone message that plays when a patient is on hold) to the practices.

The team of 0.25 FTE analyst, 0.25 FTE trainer, and 0.5 FTE programmer started with a four-month pilot in three primary-care clinics. After we assessed the pilots—based on implementation team observations and feedback from patient and staff focus groups—the team implemented the remaining 40 primary care practices sites over a 4-month period.

Since the patient EHR was the last phase of our outpatient EHR implementation, practice personnel were already familiar with the EHR's inbasket and messaging capabilities. They only needed to learn the patient sign-up process and how to triage e-messages. Training consisted of a one-hour session, followed by an afternoon of shadowing support. We also provided a Web site with FAQ's and tips.

Implementation Problems

- Initially, we required an office visit for patient enrollment. As the implementation progressed, it became clear that we needed an equally secure, but much more efficient, method for patient enrollment. Internal legal and information-security review indicated that well-designed online enrollment is acceptably secure. Patients enroll on-line by submitting personal identifying information that is already on file in the EHR (e.g., social security number, date of birth, medical record number) so that we can confirm their identity. Once identity has been established, a single-use temporary password is generated. This code is mailed (via U.S. mail) to the patient's address recorded in the EHR. This mailing provides confirmation of the application's identity by a method distinct from the online application process (i.e., "out-of-band" confirmation). When the patient logs in with the temporary password, she must provide additional identifying information to complete her registration.
- *Temporary Password Length:* Originally the temporary password was required by the EHR vendor to be 25-characters long. Patients told us this was a significant deterrent to activating their account. The vendor has reduced the required length of the password.
- *Temporary Password Expiration:* Originally, the temporary password expired in 14 days. Many patients told us that the time was too short (confirming the Help Desk's impression that 30–35% of patient calls were triggered by this problem). In response, we extended the time limit to 60 days. We also send every new registrant an e-mail reminding them how to sign-on. Finally, we send a follow-up e-mail if the patient has not signed on within 30 days. This change by itself has not resulted in an increase in the rate of patients who sign on to the patient EHR after registering for it (58%). We believe that the shorter temporary password (which we have not had time to implement) is critical to improving this rate.
- *Unanswered e-messages:* Early on, patients reported that some physicians did not return e-messages. One reason for this may be that early in the implementation physicians receive few enough e-messages that they simply forget how to reply. To address this, we changed the EHR to make replying to patient e-messages easier. We also provided refresher training throughout all our practices. In addition, executive physicians enlisted practice leaders to create incentives for physicians to answer patient e-messages. Finally, we published interviews with skillful physician users of the patient EHR in our internal print and online newsletters to spread the word that e-messaging can be a timesaver if it is used effectively.

Proxy Access

Our initial implementation of the patient EHR restricted access to adult patients. However, focus groups conducted after the initial implementations revealed that patients were sharing their IDs and passwords with their spouses and adult children in order to enable them help them manage their care. While this sharing is beyond our control, we need to be able to identify the sender of messages. Patients can now give proxy access, which allows others to access their EHR and e-messaging, on their behalf, with the correspondent identified.

Pediatric Access

Pediatric proxy access provides parents and minor children joint access to the child's EHR and e-messaging capabilities. This has the potential to engage the child more effectively in self-care of chronic diseases, such as asthma and obesity. It also gives parents the convenience of (for example) printing their child's immunization record rather than having to make a trip to the doctor's office to get a copy.

First, an interdisciplinary team of IT, clinical operations, legal, information-security, and medical records personnel reviewed our current policies and procedures, state law, and national patient confidentiality regulations (HIPAA) relating to access and release of pediatric information.

Listed below are some of the questions that we asked and answers we gave. Your questions and answers will depend critically on your state's laws and regulations, on your CDO's culture, and on your surrounding community's shared values.

- Who has the legal right to access the patient record?
  We concluded that children over 14, parents of children under age 14 (without the child's consent), and parents of children age 14–18 (with the child's consent) have the right to access the child's record.
- How is a parent defined?
  We define a parent as legal guardian of a minor, including divorced parents who retain parental rights.
- Whose signatures are required on authorization forms?
  Children aged 14–18 and their parents.
- Who receives E-mail alerts?
  The patient and all parents and legal guardians.
- How shall family conflicts (e.g., between estranged parents) over access to a minor's record be addressed?
  If parents dispute each other's access to the child's EHR, or if the parent(s) and child dispute each other's access, all access is revoked. (Printed copies of the patient's record continue to be available through the medical records department).

Physician Concerns

Some physicians were concerned about the possibility that they might have to referee disputes between parents and patients, or that minor patients simply might not bring sensitive problems to their doctor's attention for fear of a parent seeing the diagnosis in the patient's EHR (or wondering why the child suddenly revoked the parent's access). Clinical leaders and physicians on our feedback groups concluded that, in our communities, this risk was much less than the benefits many children and parents would receive from accessing children's records.

Practice Work Loads

Our approach to pediatric access requires multiple authorizations forms. While some practices managed this easily, others found that it added unacceptably to the support staff's work. For example, since the parent of a minor may not be a patient of the organization, front office personnel must collect and enter demographic information on the parent and create a unique medical record number for them.

Pediatric access is revoked when:

- A parent or minor (regardless of age) requests it.
- A physician determines that revocation is in the patient's best interest.
- A minor turns 18 years old.
- A minor is pregnant, or has been pregnant or married.
- A minor is declared emancipated by a judge (usually on the basis of living independently from his parents).
- Parental access is disputed by either a parent or the child.

Outcomes

Ross' summary of the available research is consistent with our experience thus far: "Overall, studies suggest the potential for modest benefits (for instance, in enhancing doctor-patient communication). Risks (for instance, increasing patient worry or confusion) appear to be minimal in medical patients" (5).

Our users are 59% female (as is our general practice population). Forty-nine percent of users are between the ages of 46 and 64; 18% are over 65 (see Table 19.1).

TABLE 19.1. Patient EHR Use by Age: Comparison of Users and Nonusers.

	Users $n = 4,245$ Age*	Non-users $n = 281,517$
18–30	7%	20%
31–45	27%	25%
46–64	49%	30%
65+	18%	25%
	Sex	
Female	58.6%	57.3%
Male	41.4%	42.7%
Clinic visits during the 9 months pre-implementation	3.48	2.58

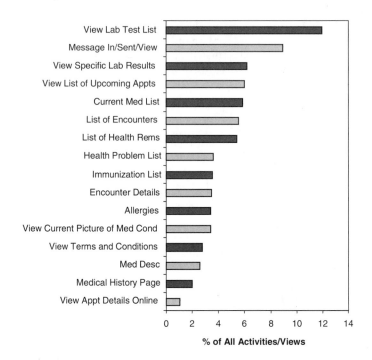

*Other poorly defined activities were each responsible for less than 1% of patient activity.

FIGURE 19.2. Most common activities/views.

Those who became active users had more office visits on average in the six months prior to enrollment than did registrants who never signed on (3.5 vs. 2.6).

Users find the patient EHR easy to use, accurate and helpful. They strongly agree that they would choose a physician based on the availability of such a service (unpublished data). In early 2004, with 8,000 users signed onto the system, we were handling 2,000 annualized prescription renewals and 2,200 appointment requests through the system.

As Figure 19.2 indicates, the most frequent uses of the site are for viewing lab test results, messaging, and viewing upcoming appointments.

Practice Efficiency

Staff feedback sessions, confidential interviews, and survey questionnaires do not reveal any effect on the workload of physicians or staff (although, in early 2004, none of our practices had more than five percent of patients using the patient EHR). E-messages appear to have replaced phone calls rather than accounting for new messaging traffic.

Production Support

Supporting a patient EHR efficiently requires these elements: information security applications and practices; fast, reliable hardware and network; and customer support. While single sign-on is not required, it does make using the patient EHR more convenient for patients to use and for our technical team to administer.

We will limit our discussion to topics that might not be immediately apparent to an experienced technical support team.

Information Security

Information security is a *sine qua non* of providing confidential patient information over the Internet. The first link in the chain of security is to confirm that none of the applications that make up the patient Web portal (which provides entry to the patient EHR) endangers the production EHR or other information systems that are critical to patient safety and core business processes. To avoid corrupting or destabilizing the production EHR, we implemented a shadow copy of the EHR and use that shadow copy to provide data to the patient EHR. Figure 19.3 illustrates the one-way feed from the production EHR to the shadow. This one-way connection makes an up-to-date copy of the EHR available to patients (and external physicians), while insulating the production EHR from the patient EHR's network traffic and possible data corruption.

The second link is a robust system for confirming the identity of users and granting them appropriate access to the various applications (including the patient EHR) that

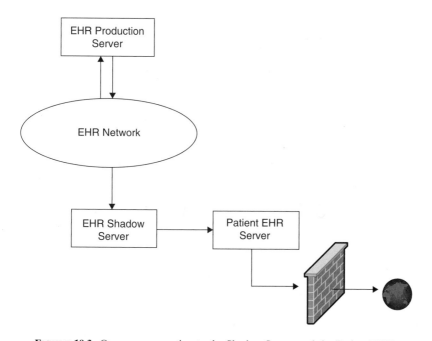

FIGURE 19.3. One-way connection to the Shadow Server and the Patient EHR.

make up the patient Web portal. To manage these functions for hundreds of thousands of projected users, we chose a software product that specializes in Web-based identity and access management (IAM), RSA ClearTrust®. The benefits of such a system include:

- Reliable identification of users
- Convenient sign-on for users: Users receive access to every appropriate application with a single sign-on (one ID and password).
- Efficient administration: The single Web security system manages access to all of the organization's Web resources for all of our customers, both internal and external.
- Simplified user-account management: Shared roles, e.g., "patient" or "external physician," give users access to appropriate applications and services while minimizing administration costs.
- Delegated administration of user accounts.
- Detection of attempts at unauthorized access and automated staff notification and/or preventive action
- Centralized logging of all patient, clinician and administrative actions

The third link in information security is a secure (128-bit encrypted) messaging interface between patients and their doctor's practices. To achieve this level of security, patients' creation of messages and reading of the replies is performed on our secure servers exclusively. Only a notification that a message is available crosses the Internet or enters the patient's e-mail system (at home, at work or elsewhere).

Fourth, giving large numbers of external users access to clinical information systems requires a careful review of data security policies. For example, forced password expiration is not likely to be acceptable to patients. Using advice from information security consultants, our own research on industry best practices, and our existing security policies, we created the following policies:

- **Remote access:** Patient-related messages and information shall receive 128-bit encryption for transmission over the Internet.
- **User ID:** ID's shall be unique. They shall never be reused or reassigned to another user. They shall have between three and 18 characters. The patient may choose the ID.
- **Password:** Passwords shall be between five and 18 characters long, with at least one numeric and one alphabetic character. The patient may select the password (with the exception of 25,000 easily guessed passwords). The password shall not expire automatically, but the patient may change it at any time. The password shall be disabled after three invalid attempts to sign-on. The password shall not be transmitted via phone or unsecured e-mail. It shall not be viewable by Geisinger employees.
- **Session Log-outs:** Sessions shall time out after 30 minutes of inactivity. The maximum active session length shall be eight hours.
- **Registration:** Registration of a new user shall include a single-use, temporary password and an out-of-band element (such as mailing the temporary access code to the patient's previously recorded home address by U.S. mail).
- **Password Reset Self-Service:** The patient may reset their password online by successfully answering a previously recorded challenge question. A confirmation letter regarding this password reset is sent by U.S. Mail to the patient's home address contained in the EHR database (to alert the patient of any unauthorized password change).

Single Sign-On (SSO)

For online services to be useful to patients, they must be easy to access. Single sign-on (SSO) gives patients access to many functions (their EHR, clinical messaging, online billing inquiries, online education) using a single ID and password. SSO provides a way to incorporate new applications and services into a patient (or other) EHR efficiently and seamlessly.

Integrating existing systems (some of which are not SSO-capable) into an SSO system is a challenge. Substantial reprogramming of our Web applications, careful planning with our IAM and EHR vendors, and extensive testing were necessary. We then had to help patients move from the first version of the patient EHR to the upgraded version that supported SSO. If feasible, the best practice is to implement SSO with the initial release of the patient EHR.

Customer Support

As patient EHR use grows, new users may be less knowledgeable about computers than were the early adopters—and less willing to spend time learning how the patient EHR works. The patient EHR needs to be very easy to use if we are to achieve our goals of improving patients' experience of healthcare while improving efficiency. In addition, it will need efficient support mechanisms.

Since this will often be your organization's first attempt to provide IT support directly to external customers, there will be many unknowns. For example, how many calls can we expect? Who will answer the calls? How long will each call take to answer? To whom will calls be triaged? Will patient calls be included in the support tracking system?

Initially, our patient EHR implementation team handled patient calls. This enabled the team to understand the types of questions we would receive and develop appropriate responses. During this pilot we learned that:

- Many patients were not aware of how to upgrade their Web browser to benefit from 128-bit encryption. We created a Web page with "Frequently Asked Questions (FAQ)" explaining encryption. The page includes a link to another Web site where users can check their Web browser's ability to support 128-bit encryption. Finally, we added links to the Microsoft® and Netscape® sites where users can update their Web browsers.
- Expired Temporary Passwords: One of the most frequent reasons for support calls was the forced expiration of the temporary password before the patient was ready to register. Delaying the temporary password's expiration has largely eliminated this reason for calls.
- Forgotten IDs and Passwords: This was the single most frequent reason for calls. Enabling patients to reset their passwords online has reduced total time spent on user support by about 50%.

Availability

Most patient users call for help during evenings and weekends—times when internal needs for Help-Desk support are low and staff availability is very limited (second shift) or unavailable except for emergencies (third shift).

TABLE 19.2. Patient-Patient EHR Related Use of the Help Desk.

	Calls	% of Total Users	Total Minutes	Minutes per Call	Total Users
Apr-03	97	2.2	230	2	4484
Jun-03	92	1.8	216	2	5251
Aug-03	48	0.8	95	2	6002
Oct-03	72	1.0	168	2	6898
Dec-03	34	0.46	88	3	7381
Feb-04	61	0.73	140	2	8366
Apr-04	101	1.0	454	5	10064
Jun-04	88	0.74	283	3	11929

After the patient-EHR team completed its analysis and design of the user support system and a Web-based tool that provides the Help Desk personnel the information they need to answer most questions, we transferred the responsibility of taking the patient calls (on first and second shift) to the general IT Help Desk. Calls that cannot be handled by the second-shift Help Desk person and calls that come in on third shift go to a voice mailbox monitored by the patient-EHR team. As Table 19.2 shows, demand on the Help Desk has decreased while the number of active users has increased sharply, suggesting that our efforts to make the patient EHR easier to use and to provide effective online help have been effective.

Summary

Providing patients access to their EHR and e-messaging to their doctor's practice delights a growing number of customers and shows signs of creating practice efficiencies. If the patient EHR is a module of the core EHR, technical set-up and clinician training needs are modest.

References

1. James H, Newcomer & Smiljanich PA. Former Fox News TV Producer Sues Major Pharmaceutical Company And NY Clinic Over Ineffective Hepatitis A Vaccine, 2003. http://www.forrelease.com/D20030514/flw024.P2.05142003161018.17746.html
2. Committee on Quality of Health Care in America IOM. Crossing the Quality Chasm: A New Health System for the 21st Century. Washington, DC: National Academy Press; 2001.
3. Coombes A. Retired, and more wired: Older Americans ramp up Internet use; site designers have yet to catch up, 2003. http://cbs.marketwatch.com/news/story.asp?guid=%7BE5A6935D-1B46-4252-B07B-A58C143ADC50%7D&siteid=google&dist=google
4. Taylor H, Leitman R. Patient/Physician Online Communication: Many patients want it, would pay for it, and it would influence their choice of doctors and health plans. Harris Interactive; 2002.
5. Ross SE, Lin C-T. The Effects of Promoting Patient Access to Medical Records: A Review. *J Am Med Informatics* 2003;10:129–38.

20
Extending EHR Access to External Physicians

JOAN E. TOPPER and KATHLEEN M. DEAN

Introduction

One of the most important potential benefits of an EHR is improved communication among providers, outside as well as inside the organization. This chapter presents our experience with a variety of methods for extending EHR access to affiliated providers, whom we define as any provider who serves on the staff of our community hospital, who refers patients to us, or to whom we refer patients.

In 2000, a survey of affiliated physicians indicated that more timely and complete clinical communication is one of their three most important criteria for referring patients to another CDO. This prompted us to look for ways to extend EHR access to them. While existing communication channels (e.g., U.S. mail, fax, telephone, face-to-face conversations) are each useful, the EHR and Web applications can deliver patient information to affiliated providers more rapidly, securely, reliably, and cost effectively.

We have developed three main approaches to providing information to affiliated providers. First, we created a Web portal containing episode-specific information. Next, we provided affiliates access to the complete EHR. Most recently, we automated the routing of electronic and transcribed patient encounter documentation.

Organization

To lead this effort, we hired an e-Health Director with a mandate from executive leadership to coordinate the efforts of clinical operations, marketing and IT. To gain guidance and support, the director created a steering committee comprised of a vice-president of clinical operations, the Director of marketing, the CIO, the CMIO, the Director of EHR projects, the Director of Web Services, and the Director of Patient Safety.

Needs Assessment

A 2000 survey indicated that these are the six online services that are most attractive to our affiliated physicians:

1. Access to the patient's EHR
2. Access to electronic medical reference information

3. Access to continuing medical education (CME) courses
4. Automatic notification of significant patient events (e.g., discharge summaries)
5. Easier communication with Geisinger physicians
6. Referral appointment scheduling

Phase 1: General Information

In May 2001, we implemented the first phase of the e-health project, an affiliated-physician section on our external Web site (http://www.geisinger.org).

The section contained several features:

- CME information
- Schedules of specialists' availability at outreach clinics
- Patient education materials
- Healthcare news
- Information about Geisinger clinical services

As we expected from the survey, these resources did not provide enough value to motivate much use (about 200 site visits a month).

Phase 2: Event-Based Information Reporting

Next, we added core information (date of admission, patient location, demographics, insurance, date of discharge and discharge summary) on patients seen at a Geisinger clinical facility in the last 90 days. Software scans the EHR database each night for new patient information (primarily office visits or hospitalizations) and posts it to the secure Web account of the patient's referring and primary-care physicians. While this section of the portal does not provide all of the information in the patient's EHR, affiliated physicians find it useful—particularly since it streamlines existing paper workflows, rather than requiring new ones.

Affiliated providers report these benefits:

- Rapid notification of patient admission and discharges
- Simplified navigation (since only recent records are included)
- A convenient list of patients in the hospital (by provider and by practice)
- Patient consent is not needed since the provider sees only information related to care they ordered or referred the patient for.

Portal Access

The portal's target market is physicians, but it is usually the staff who access medical records to prepare them for physician use. We developed a security system that manages the access given to physicians, mid-level providers, nurses, billing clerks and other office staff.

When a physician requests access to the portal, we ask them to designate an individual (usually the office manager) as the practice's contact person. This individual is responsible for identifying other staff members who need access. Each staff member signs an individual user agreement and receives a unique ID and password that she is required to change at a set interval. (This enables us to create HIPAA-compliant records of access.) Physicians and practices agree to notify us when a staff member leaves.

If one physician in a practice has a care relationship with a patient, any authorized person from that office may access information. This allows physicians to cover each other during absences and gives office staff the access they need to coordinate care.

Phase 3: Single-Patient EHR Access

In the third phase of the project, we used one of our EHR vendor's products (EpicLink®) to provide affiliated physicians access to the full EHR of patients. We began by piloting the service in one practice in 2001.

Physician access to the entire EHR has the potential to improve patient safety (for instance, by ensuring that the patient's full medicine list is available) and healthcare efficiency (by recording that the patient's latest tetanus shot was four years ago). It also has the potential to compromise patient confidentiality (e.g., the orthopedic surgeon treating his neighbor's ankle fracture sees that the patient has a history of depression).

Because we cannot protect patient confidentiality by limiting this global access to the EHR, we require the requesting physician to send us the patient's written authorization before allowing access. These authorizations are valid for three years. (In feedback groups, patients unanimously support a longer interval, 20 years or more. As we gain more experience with privacy regulations, we plan to extend the interval.)

The requirement that each patient authorize each affiliated provider's access – particularly given the accompanying 24-48-hour delay until access activation – is a major disincentive to provider use. Most believe that since they have a direct care relationship with that patient, they should be able to access the patient's information without specific authorization. This feeling is reinforced by the fact that they receive much of the same information (test results, notes, letters) on paper without an authorization.

Since the affiliated physician access module of our EHR simply provides a secure Web-based view into the EHR, technical set-up was relatively simple. The one security issue that we needed to address was the fact that the original version of the product accessed the production EHR. Even over a secured Internet connection, this posed a small, but unacceptable risk of corrupting the EHR's database. We resolved the issue by installing a shadow server to which this application, as well as the patient-access application, is directed.

Each practice's implementation required a network generalist (see Chapter 13) to visit the practice and load the client software on all the computers that would be used to access patient records.

The practices agreed to the following conditions:

- To provide computers and connectivity to the Internet (usually a dedicated phone line).
- To use 128-bit encryption.
- To have "cookies" turned on (a requirement for the software to work).
- To sign a confidentiality agreement. Each user signs an individual use agreement, and each is assigned a unique user ID and temporary activation password.

Access to the patients' entire EHR can make locating information a challenge for inexperienced users. Physicians and their staff may need extensive (eight to 16 hours) training to use the EHR effectively. Because they use the EHR only intermittently, learning will be slow and hard to consolidate. For these reasons, many affiliated physicians prefer access to the smaller (hence, more navigable) event-based data set.

Phase 4: Streamlined Document Distribution

Streamlined document distribution is a feature we built into our EHR. When a provider finishes documenting a patient encounter in the EHR, he can invoke a screen in which to indicate providers he wants to receive copies of the note. The patient's primary-care physician and referring provider are automatically included—if that information was recorded when the patient checked in. There is also a pick-list of providers who have previously received communications regarding the patient. At the next level of generality, any provider in the region can be selected by pattern matching. Finally, a free-text box allows entering the name and address of a provider who is not presently in the database. Overnight, the application sends the note to the receiving provider's preferred address (fax, U.S. mail, or e-mail).

As usual, the technical set-up was the easiest part of the project. Verifying every regional physician's address, telephone number, fax number and preferred communication channel took hundreds of person-hours. As a next step, we are considering adding payers to the database, to streamline provider communication with them.

Information Security

We use the Web-based access-management software and methodologies described in Chapter 19, to manage access for external physicians and practices.

Physicians can access episode-based patient records and the full EHR of individual patients from their office. However, many need at home access. This requires an additional level of security: two-factor authentication. Two-factor authentication requires something the user knows (her password) and something she has (in our case, a key fob that displays a numerical password which is synchronized with the sign-on server). We use fobs provided by our IAM vendor.

Selling It

The first rule of selling is to know your audience. The CMIO presented the portal at a medical staff meeting of our community hospital, which was attended by about 30 affiliated physicians. Each attendee received a fact sheet and the opportunity to sign up at the meeting or to call and sign-up. We received only two responses. The next month, we sent a letter to the office managers of affiliated physicians' practices (with the same invitation) and signed up 50 practices in 90 days. A year later (2004), we are serving 148 practices

Keys to Success

1. Design a comprehensive security plan early and build your services consistent with that plan. Consider single sign-on software.
2. Understand affiliated providers' needs and check your understanding frequently. An internal physician advisory board can aid with this understanding, particularly if some members are (or recently were) affiliated providers.

3. Careful coordination between clinical operations, IT and Marketing is remarkably productive.
4. Remember that electronic communication is only one communication channel among many. Telephone, US mail, fax and face-to-face communication continue to be the preferred channels for many providers. Give them information the way they want it. And remember that preferences will be changing rapidly over the next decade.

Part Four
Summary and Prospects

21
Summary and Prospects

JAMES M. WALKER

Implementing an EHR is one of the largest and most complex projects a CDO can undertake. More than that, it presents your organization (large or small) with an opportunity to re-think and re-design the ways you do business. It necessitates identifying all your customers, internal and external. It requires an intensified focus on cooperation among work groups (e.g., pediatric and adult subspecialties, physicians and nurses, practices and hospitals, clinicians and administrators). It requires that the lab, pharmacy, and other services analyze their internal customers' carefully. Table 21.1 lists some of the primary process improvements the EHR has made feasible for us.

Benefits Realized

The primary benefits of the EHR are not easily quantifiable. The most telling is the fact that our physicians simply refuse to practice in new outreach clinics until the EHR is available. The convenience of accessing and adding to the patient's complete health record, combined with the confidence that comes with automated clinical decision support—such as automatic allergy and drug-interaction checking—make the EHR indispensable for clinicians who have used it longer than six months.

Similarly, our EHR has transformed clinical communication. In our practices, telephone tag—and the enormous inefficiencies it creates—is a thing of the past. It has been replaced almost entirely by electronic messaging, sent at the sender's convenience and answered at the recipient's convenience—with the patient's record automatically attached. Even hallway tag, in which physicians and nurses chase each other down to coordinate more time-sensitive patient care, has largely been replaced by e-messaging.

Other benefits of the EHR can be at least partially quantified. Examples from our experience include:

- 372,000 fewer laboratory and radiology reports printed and filed annually
- 36% reduction in outpatient lines of transcription
- 60% reduction in paper medical record chart pulls
- 33% reduction in Medicare disallowance of bills due to medical necessity edits of tests ordered
- 94% of patients find having the EHR in the exam room helpful or very helpful.
- $1,000 per physician saved annually through increased use of generic drugs
- 97% of office visits include allergy checking and documentation.
- 100% of outpatient orders include an ICD-9 code assigned by the provider.
- 90% reduction in unauthorized visits to specialists

TABLE 21.1. Processes Improved with the EHR.

Process Type	Benefits
Patient safety	Automatic, real-time drug-drug and drug-allergy checking
Care quality	Automatic, patient-specific reminders in real time Documentation standardized, searchable, readable.
Patient access	Standardized scheduling system integrated with the EMR.
Patient information access	Anytime secure access to the EHR and to practices
Clinic workflows	Simplified, standardized workflows
Information reporting	Automated reports on aggregated clinical data
Remote access	To clinical and administrative information
Digital radiology	Remote, real-time access to most images
Outpatient quality Measurement	Automated tracking of pharmacy and ER use and patient access
Billing	Clinician linkage of orders with diagnoses
	Automatic medical necessity checking

Next Steps

Although our outpatient implementation is complete and our inpatient implementation is well underway, we are only at the beginning of using the EHR to transform the ways we provide healthcare. These are some of the next steps we have identified:

- *Explicit Goals and Measures:* We are becoming more thorough about assessing needs and defining goals—to assure congruence between EHR projects and organizational strategies—and particularly about pre-defining the measures by which we check our progress toward those goals. As goals are reached, we will need to define new ones for the next phase of improvement. When goals are missed, we analyze both the failure and the goal and make the changes needed to accomplish the goal (or a revised goal). Even a change as apparently simple as decreasing chart pulls requires active management.
- *Operational Leadership:* Clinical and administrative leaders are increasingly leading EHR projects, both through their roles on oversight and feedback committees and by taking responsibility for identifying new business initiatives that the EHR can support. A particularly effective example is the streamlined document distribution discussed in Chapter 20, which was conceived by a task force working on improving our relationships with referring physicians. The task force identified a need for more rapid communication with referring physicians and the EHR team was able to customize the EHR to help meet the need.
- *Integrated Workflows:* One of the chief virtues of an EHR based on a single database is its potential to support seamless care across the spectrum of care, from home to outpatient, inpatient, and long-term care. To achieve this potential will require painstaking analysis and process re-design by all CDOs and equally painstaking efforts on the part of EHR vendors. The solutions to even basic needs—such as complete accounting for the changes made in a patient's medicines in the transition from outpatient to inpatient care and back—are in the early developmental stages.
- *Standardized Implementations:* If the EHR is to be implemented effectively by thousands of American CDOs over the next decade, we will need to develop standardized implementation methodologies that are efficient enough that community hospitals, physician practices, and their patients can benefit from using a high-performance EHR (i.e., one that is capable of provider order entry and real-time

decision support, that is accompanied by appropriate workflows and that is supported by the communications capabilities discussed in Chapters 20 and 21. We and other organizations are developing these methodologies, but careful research is needed to identify the critical challenges to widespread implementation and demonstrate how to overcome them.

- *EHR Tool Development:* One enabler of widespread EHR implementation will be the development of high-efficiency, validated, shareable EHR tools (e.g., note templates and order sets). While many tools have been built, we need to standardize their construction, assessment, and maintenance. We need to set them in the context of proven change methodologies (1, 2). We need to know more about the factors that lead to and discourage their use (3).

- *Use of the Patient EHR for Patient Interview and Education:* Patients' access to secure e-messaging has the potential to help us address critical gaps in healthcare provision. For example, a substantial research literature shows that computerized patient interview is effective, especially in patients with low literacy. (4) One way patient interview could be used is suggested by Gandhi, et.al's. study which found that 8% of outpatients had an ameliorable adverse event attributable to a newly prescribed medicine, which was not addressed due to the patient not reporting the symptoms to the physician or the physician's failure to respond to the symptoms. (5) Using currently available technology, a software utility could scan the EHR for new prescriptions and send patients an electronic (or telephoned or mailed) questionnaire one week after the prescription inquiring about adverse effects and relaying any positive results to the prescribing provider (along with management suggestions).

- *Careful Studies of the Effectiveness of the EHR on Efficiency and Quality:* Finally, we need to perform real-world effectiveness studies of production EHRs in routine clinical use. While we have clear evidence that many elements of EHRs—and the systems of care they support—work in research settings, we have little knowledge of the incremental contribution each may make in other settings (e.g., healthcare systems, community hospitals, large and small independent provider groups). We need this information to choose among multiple potentially useful implementation options.

References

1. Davis DA. Translating guidelines into practice: A systematic review of theoretic concepts, practical experience and research evidence in the adoption of clinical practice guidelines. *Can Med Assoc J* 1997;157:408–416.
2. Brook RH, Williams K. Quality assurance today and tomorrow: forecast for the future. *Ann Intern Med* 1976;85:809.
3. Flottorp S, Oxman AD, Håvelsrud K. Cluster randomised controlled trial of tailored interventions to improve the management of urinary tract infections in women and sore throat. *Br Med J* 2002;325:367.
4. Campbell MK. What patients need beyond more accessible information. AMIA Spring Congress: Bridging the Digital Divide–Informatics and Vulnerable Populations. Philadelphia; 2003.
5. Gandhi T, Weingart S, Borus J, Leape LL, Bates DW. Adverse Drug Events in Ambulatory Care. *New Engl J Med* 2003:348;1556.

Appendices

Appendix 1

The following summary identifies the key system-wide policy decisions which provided the framework for regional implementation of the CPR.

Security

1. Access to medical records should be on a need to know basis. Only those providers and employees with a clear need to view patient specific information should have access. Access should be restricted based on job description—e.g., a physician has different access than a secretary. The present technology does not yet provide the tools to guarantee this. However, policy should be clear that one should only seek access when and where it is necessary as part of one's legitimate job function.
2. An ongoing audit trail must be created of all transactions and accesses to the system. Random and systematic review of the audit trail should be accomplished regularly to test compliance with confidentiality policies.
3. Provisions for restricted visit types (HIV, Drug and Alcohol Treatment, Mental Health) and restricted records (VIPs, employees, etc.) are necessary. Access for those not already providing direct care should be via "break the glass" access creating an audit trail.
4. The security policy strictly prohibits sharing of passwords or using another person's password. Passwords must be changed every 6 months.
5. Violations of the security/confidentiality policy *be* pursued by supervisors and Human Resources.
6. Access to the system shall be immediately revoked upon employee termination.

Utilization Management

1. Associating all services and orders with an encounter diagnosis/symptom in an accurate and consistent fashion is an organizational expectation of all providers.
2. Every patient shall have an identified Primary Care Provider (PCP).
3. Problem list maintenance is the ultimate responsibility of the PCP.
4. Accurate and consistent coding of encounter diagnoses by the provider is an organizational expectation.

Orders

1. Order entry will be performed directly by the provider and completed prior to check-out for an office visit.
2. Standardized order requisitions will be established for the system.
3. All orders (procedures, medications, referrals, ancillary testing, etc.) must be associated with an appropriate diagnosis.
4. Each site will develop specific workflow rules regarding ordering procedures and corresponding co-sign requirements.
5. Orders from the system shall be electronically interfaced with order receiving departments (for example, the Radiology Information System (RIS) and the Laboratory Information System (LIS)).
6. Processes for order cancellation will be defined at a system level. The flow of information will be coordinated between the EHR and the interfaced ancillary systems.

Scheduling

1. The needs of the patient are always the top priority in the scheduling process.
2. Cadence will be implemented based upon a 3-tier model for scheduling.
   - Primary Care
   - Specialty Departments
   - Call Center

   This three-tiered model enables clinics to schedule any and all appointments for the patient at the point of service. Utilizing a rules-based functionality, the primary care sites will be able to schedule specialty appointments for the patient. If however, the primary care site staff would be unsuccessful in obtaining the right day, time, provider, etc., then the specific specialty department would be able to assist in scheduling. Depending on staffing needs, the specialty tier would be staffed by reallocating existing central appointments to the specialty department. The remaining centralized core of schedulers would be integrated with the call center and are the third tier "super schedulers". They address those situations where the number of appointments and sequencing of appointments is complex and time consuming.
3. Patient access, provider availability, and effective utilization of provider time will be actively managed through department/work unit template development.

Referral Authorization

1. There shall be one physician who manages referrals for each patient. This will be the patient's assigned primary care provider (PCP).
2. The referral status of a consult visit ordered by a PCP is automatically authorized.
3. The referral status of a consult visit ordered by a specialist is also automatically authorized given the following caveats:
   - Subject to PCP review/denial via electronic notification
   - Requests for additional visits **or** consults with another specialist must be related to the condition/problem noted on the original consult from the PCP.
4. If the PCP denies the consult request, an automatic message is returned to the specialist with the reason for denial. Additionally, an automatic message is sent to the

PCP's support staff indicating the appropriate patient follow-up activity, e.g. call patient, schedule appointment, etc.

5. The PCP is responsible for timely (within 24 business hours) review of electronic referral request messages residing in his/her In-Basket.

Note: This design must be understood in the context of 1995. The GHS assumed financial risk for a large population (the health plan membership). There were no contracts with other managed care organizations at the time. This design has been modified over time.

Results Reporting

1. The CPR will be established as the clinical data base for all medical results data. Although the system is initially focused on outpatient practices, inpatient data is also included.
2. Data will be transferred electronically from ancillary systems, such as lab, radiology, EKG and distinguish preliminary from final results. The use of handwritten results will be phased out over time.
3. Adjunct technologies will be used to fill data gaps and provide needed information: e.g., digital cameras for patient photographs, scanners for paper documents which cannot be accessed electronically, and links to other systems such as medical imaging systems.
4. Paper reports will be eliminated when access to the electronic report is available.

Point of Service/Billing

Appointment Scheduling

1. Pre-registration is performed at this time, and could therefore qualify the patient for express registration at appointment check-in.
2. Schedulers will verify insurance information (confirm major payor category) and provide co-pay and balance due reminders.
3. Patient demographics will be verified and insurance benefit coverage estimates will be available.
4. Schedulers will link the appropriate referral to the visit.

Patient Check-In

1. The scheduling system will be consistently used to monitor patient wait times.
2. The computer system will guide the staff through the required steps for the two types of registration: Express Registration or Full Registration.
3. This registration process will be used consistently across the organization. A key enable or is an effective training and credentialing program.

Patient Check-Out

1. The provider completes orders, diagnoses, and associations prior to patient check-out.

2. The goal of check-out is to provide the patient with a summary of their visit, including charge information, and to collect patient obligations. Ultimately, the vision includes real time adjudication with insurance carriers.
3. Day-of-service cash collections will be pursued for patient obligations for today's visit, today-for-today ancillaries, and past-due balances.
4. Ancillaries will pursue day-of-service cash collection for ancillary-only visits and will therefore require cash drawer functionality.
5. Payments collected at the point of service will be posted by front office staff.
6. The check-out process will also include scheduling today-for-today and future appointments.

Benefits Engine

A benefits engine with payor and coverage information will provide patients and clinicians with coverage information prior to the appointment and at the point of service.

Appendix 2
Physician Reporting and Digital Storage System Needs Assessment— Endoscopy Suite

1 Introduction

The needs assessment for the system-wide software solution for physician reporting and digital storage system in the Endoscopy Suite represents one of several steps taken to provide Geisinger Health System (GHS) with a software solution able to meet its business requirements and long-term objectives. Specifically, the goal of this needs assessment is to meet the GHS vision of growth by increasing the throughput of procedures completed in the Endoscopy Suite. This document provides an explanation of the functions that are proposed for implementation in the new system. The functionality requirements are: input of data, image capture and storage, retrieval, and reporting capabilities for the Endoscopy Suite procedure data.

2 Current Methods and Procedures

2.1 Overview

The Endoscopy Suite performs procedures on adults and pediatric patients. For the year 2001, the total procedures completed in the Endoscopy suite were: Adult procedures—5400, Flex Sigmoidoscopy—1400, and Pediatrics procedures—750. The patients, who include inpatients and outpatients, are referred from both Geisinger and non-Geisinger physicians. Occasionally, patients are transferred from Geisinger Wyoming Valley (GWV) and admitted as inpatients at Geisinger Medical Center (GMC). For an overview of the Endoscopy Suite workflow, refer to attachment A.

There are four major procedures, which include Colonoscopy, Upper Endoscopy (EGD), Endoscopic Retrograde Cholangiopancreatitogram (ERCP), and Flexible Sigmoidoscopy. In addition, the physician can complete several sub-procedures for one billing encounter.

Recently, the Endoscopy Suite expanded the procedure area for a total of five procedure rooms, four adult and one pediatric. Future expansion includes additional physicians to perform procedures, one adult and two pediatric physicians. Within six months, the department will perform an endoscopic treatment for reflux disease (Stretta Procedure).

2.2 Nurse/Technician Documentation

The nurse and technician document on the Endoscopy Flow Sheet (refer to attachments B and C). The flow sheet includes all the documentation from pre-procedure assessment to discharge instructions. It is available for update during the procedures to document vital signs and patient's progress. The nurse documents all the medications given in the Endoscopy Suite, as ordered by the physician, on the Outpatient Medication Sheet. In addition, the nurse completes the Conscious Sedation Record when the patient is sedated. During the procedure the images are captured from the clinical equipment and printed to photo paper.

For pediatric patients, the pre-assessment is completed and prep initiated in the pediatric clinic prior to the endoscopy procedure. For adult patients, Carelink mails the patient instructions and prep prescriptions to the patient. The patient chooses which prep to use and completes the prep at home. Prior to the procedure, the Endosopy-Suite nurse completes the pre-procedure assessment.

2.3 Physician Documentation

On average, the physician documentation process for each patient involves twelve minutes of post procedure time. The physician hand writes the procedure report on a preprinted form and completes the post discharge instruction form. In addition, medications and additional studies are ordered when indicated. The physician determines the appropriate billing and checks the procedure codes on the service sheet.

2.4 Checkout and Discharge Procedures

Once the patient is finished with a procedure the provider decides the time period for a return appointment, if indicated. The provider completes the "Gastroenterology Procedure Follow-Up Card". This card includes the following: Patient Name, Medical Record Number (MRN), Physician, Diagnosis, Follow-Up Desired, Procedure Difficult, Barium Enema (BE), Flexible Sigmoidoscopy, Colonoscopy, Esophagogastroduodenoscopy (EGD), antibiotic prophylaxis needed, Anticoagulation: Yes, aspirin (ASA), Coumadin, Other, or No, Reschedule Study in: weeks, months, years, Preparation: Golytely, Visicol, Fleet1/2, Fleet Phospho-soda. This card is presented to the receptionist upon discharge of the patient. The receptionist enters all the appropriate information into the scheduling system, and the patient is placed on this wait list, also known as the recall list, awaiting an appointment. Carelink is responsible for the recall list and contacts the patient to schedule the appointment. The appointment is mailed to the patient along with an instructiom booklet for the procedure, the prep needed, and a prescription for that prep.

At the conclusion of the encounter, the receptionist files all the images from the procedure(s) in a plastic sleeve and files them along with all the documentation in the medical record. The receptionist schedules appointments in the scheduling system.

2.5 Quality Improvement (QI) Documentation

The Endospocy Suite developed an Access database to store patient information for each procedure for Q.I. reporting. Daily, the Endoscopy Suite staff enters the following information into this database: date of procedure, MRN, inpatient/outpatient status, Endoscopist, type of procedure, biopsy taken, cytology taken, frozen section biopsy taken, complications during the procedure, findings, and interventions.

The staff query the data to produce the following reports: procedures per month, procedures per Endoscopist, specific month and Endoscopist, MRN, type of procedure, interventions, complications and findings.

3 Project Goals

- Increase patient throughput by minimizing physician documentation time.
- Ensure maximum reimbursement through proper documentation and determination of billing codes electronically.
- Acquire and store images digitally.
- Increase referring physician satisfaction with image-enhanced reports.
- Create reports using discreet fields that are user-friendly and easily customized without Information Technology support.
- Interface the image storage and reporting system with equipment in the Endoscopy Suite.
- Send ADT data to the image storage and reporting system.
- Send reports to the EHR with a link to images in the image storage and report system.
- Interface results using a single system to serve multiple departments, if the image storage and report system has additional modules.
- Provide patient education materials.
- Streamline the quality-improvement process.

4 Assumptions

The needs assessment is based on the following assumptions:

- The billing process will remain the same.
- Nurses will continue to document using the current record and will not document in the new system (refer to attachments B and C). Electronic nursing documentation will be revisited when additional solutions are available for other departments (i.e. intensive care and operating room).
- The "Recall List" is considered out of the scope of the project. The "Recall list" is stored in the scheduling system on the wait list, which includes patient demographics, procedure, and return appointment time. In addition, there are comments regarding a previous procedure such as complications, sedation, and antibiotics given.
- Since images are currently stored on paper, there will not be a historical load of images.
- The scheduling, patient education, and prep that are completed prior to the procedure will remain the same.
- The staff in the Endoscopy Suite will use the EHR as read only access.
- One system will meet the needs of all patients (adult pediatric, inpatient, and outpatient).
- One of the Endoscopy Suite staff will be assigned the system administrator responsibilities along with a back up administrator from IT.
- The IT Technical Analyst will provide purchase orders for hardware and software per the specifications provided by the vendor.
- Geisinger Facilities will install the cabling required to run the application.

5 Functional Requirements

5.1 Description

An assessment was completed in the Endoscopy Suite to determine functional needs of an application to meet the goals of this project.

5.2 Application

The application will include:

- Electronic generation of the appropriate CPT-4 and ICD-9 codes for each procedure, including sub-procedures, to assure accurate billing.
- The capability to update CPT-4 and ICD-9 codes to match the billing system (ability to update outside of an upgrade process).
- Calculation of an age in years for adult patients; and days, weeks, and months, for pediatric patients- to accommodate both adult and pediatric procedures.
- Upload of the standard provider database along with routine updates to the application database for interface filing.
- User-friendly, customizable pull-down menus for intuitive entry of data.
- Customized lists are automatically maintained as application upgrades are applied to ensure continuity of user defined data.
- A medication list that can be maintained by department, which includes the specific adult and pediatric dosages for each medication.
- The ability to deactivate items on lists that are not required while maintaining the items for historical purposes, to prevent users from selecting invalid data while maintaining previous data for reporting.
- A searchable field that can be customized to add equipment serial numbers and lot numbers to provide query functions for tracking and reporting of equipment.
- A field that can link to a table that includes additional information equipment specifications.
- The ability to keep multiple cases open at one workstation until all information is completed, so that the staff can move from case to case without finalizing previous patients.
- The ability to read non-confirmed reports at all workstations that run the application, to provide the physician with several access modes.
- The ability to open a report simultaneously at multiple workstations, allowing one user write access and others read only access.
- Patient identification that is visible on the screen to ensure that the staff document on the correct patient.
- A field to define patient type (inpatient and outpatient) to classify patients for reporting, billing, and interface transactions.
- The ability to identify different equipment when the equipment is swapped out in the procedure room to ensure accurate documentation of serial and lot numbers.
- Fields to define participants, which include technicians, nurses, fellows, and staff physicians to use for documentation and reporting.
- An audit trail to track access and modifications to ensure information security and confidentiality.
- Ongoing development for new procedures and the ability to retrofit to past revisions to maintain all procedure data in one system.
- The ability to compartmentalize additional department modules and limit access by department, to ensure confidentiality of patient data.

5.3 Image Capture and Storage

- The ability to capture all images and indicate which images to retain for future reference.
- The ability to select multiple images, up to a maximum of 10, to include on the pro-cedure report (for sharing information with referring physicians).
- Image retrieval from previous procedures to incorporate in the new pocedure (to demonstrate whether the patient's condition is improving or deteriorating).
- The ability to print to networked laser or local color printers to give the physician the option to print a higher quality image or less expensive image to give to the patient.
- Prompt (sub-second) response time for retrieving images stored on the server to maximize physician efficiency.
- The ability to import selected electronic images to the image storage and reporting system from other applications, such as the Given Endoscopic Capsule, to maintain one image repository for the Endoscopy Suite.

5.4 Procedure Reporting

The application will include:

- A final report that lists all CPT and ICD-9 codes relevant to the procedure, to assist physician with billing.
- The ability to revise CPT and ICD-9 codes in the system to maintain up to date clas-sification and reimbursement codes.
- Customized reports for the four core procedures listed above in the Current Proce-dures and Methods section. Each core procedure has multiple sub-procedures; pro-cedures; the system must supply a reporting tool for each.
- The ability to add/edit data to a confirmed report (report will create a parent/child relationship for history of changes).
- Prompt (sub-second) response time for retrieving reports stored on the server to maximize physician efficiency.

5.5 QI/Research

The application will include:

- A searchable database including but not limited to the following fields:
  - Physician
  - Procedure
  - Complications
  - Diagnoses
- The ability to generate reports which can be customized to fit the needs of referring physicians.
- The ability to define outcome measures predetermined by the Endoscopy Suite, such as:
  - Quality and Outcomes
    - Endoscopic perforation rate of less than 0.1%.
    - Ninety-day readmission rate.
    - Clinical trial participation.

- Development of CME materials, practice guidelines, and EHR-based screening algorithms.

5.6 Patient Education

The application will include dischange instructions that can be customized by patient, procedure, physician, patient age, or patient type (inpatient & outpatient). The instructions must be printable and retained electronically.

5.7 Capacity Limits

The application and/or archive servers will include:

- The ability to store reports and images to comply with federally mandated patient-record retention requirements.
- The ability to purge information based on the age of the patient when the procedure was completed, to comply with mandated record-retention requirements.

5.8 Backup/Archive Data

The application will include:

- A RAID away that will include a copy of the primary hard drive that can be swapped into production if the primary drive is corrupted.
- The ability to send data to a mirrored server located at a remote site to ensure prompt access to the system when the primary server is down.
- The ability to archive data in a format that will be retrievable within five minutes.
- The ability to store images in the system-wide repository (using the storage area network (SAN)).
- The ability to archive images to the PACS system with the image pointer transferred from this application to PACS.

5.9 Network Compatibility

The digital image and reporting system must conform to the standards set forth in attachment D.

5.10 Test Environment

The application will include a non-production environment in which to test new updates and how they interact with existing interfaces.

5.11 Longitudinal Solution

The application will:

- Capture images from remote sites, to maintain a single, central repository.
- Import images that are located at one site to complete a study performed at another site.

- Store images on a portable computer and manually download the images to the image storage and archive system, enabling the staff to use the system during network downtimes.
- Upload images from previous procedures to the portable computer for comparison.

5.12 Training

The training agreement will include:

- System administration training.
- On site "go live" training during implementation.
- Follow up training after implementation.

5.13 Support

The support agreement will include:

- Primary level of support from vendor.
- Support from vendor, who will work with the Server Management Team to assist with data recovery.
- Support from the vendor during scheduled and unscheduled downtimes to assist with technical issues.

5.14 Software Upgrades

Upgrades to software will include:

- Interface testing in a non-production environment before implementation in the production environment.
- Upgrades to the interface software when required and coordination of upgrades so that there is no loss of functionality.
- Geisinger customizations are automatically maintained as application upgrades are applied.

5.15 ADT Interface

The ADT interface will:

- Conform to HL-7 standards.
- Purge patient data from the application within a specified time.
- Populate the following data fields in the reporting application:
  - Last name, first name, middle initial
  - Medical record number
  - Date of birth
  - Gender
  - Location
  - Referring physician
  - Scheduled appointment physician
  - Inpatient/outpatient indicator
  - Hospital billing number

- Allow users to choose what data to send to the image storage and reporting system.
- Allow data revision, e.g., if a procedure is completed by a second physician.
- Create error logs to assist with troubleshooting.

5.16 Results Interface

The results interface to the EHR will:

- Conform to HL-7 standards.
- Create error logs to assist in troubleshooting conflicts.
- Send the following required fields to the interface engine:
  - Last name, first name, middle initial
  - Medical record number
  - Date of birth
  - Gender
  - Clinic location
  - Referring physician
  - Confirming physician
  - Inpatient/outpatient indicator
  - Billing number
  - Field to identify a parent/child relationship
- Produce the report in the EHR that is an exact replica of the report in the image storage and reporting system.
- Merge two records for the same patient with two medical record numbers to ensure that the procedure is filed in the correct patient record.
- Update the report with accurate information and create audit trail, when a report is linked to the wrong patient.

6 Security/HIPPA Requirements

6.1 Passwords

All passwords comply with the following requirements:

- Each user ID shall be unique (and never re-used).
- Each password shall consist of five to eight characters, at least one of them a number.
- Passwords shall be changed every six months.

6.2 Data-Access Control Software

The data-access control software must comply with the following requirements:

- Passwords shall not be displayed on the screen when entered.
- Passwords shall not print on audit trails or user reports.
- After three failed attempts to enter the password, the user ID shall be suspended requiring. System administrator intervention shall be required for reactivation.
- Internal storage of passwords shall be in encrypted form.
- Violations shall be recorded in an audit log.
- Users shall create their passwords.

6.3 Audit Log

The audit log contains entries for the following (along with the user ID, date and time of access):

- Addition of any record
- Modification of any record
- Deletion of any record
- Access of any record
- Addition and modifications to patient education instructions

6.4 Logoff

Automatic logoff that is user-profile specific (a security procedure that causes an electronic session to terminate after a predetermined time of inactivity).

7 Hardware Compatibility

The application must be compatible with the Olympus and Pentax equipment used to capture images, along with third party vendor hardware that connects to the Olympus and Pentax equipment. The vendor will ensure future compatibility. In addition, the application will include the ability to:

- Download data to the application from a portable computer.
- Upload previous images to a portable computer to add to a new exam.
- Print to a networked printer and to a local printer.

8 Viability of Vendor

The following factors will be considered to estimate potential each vendors viability as a long-term partner:

- Headquarters, other locations
- Revenue
- Number of employees
- Market/Industry information
- Organization Structure
- Annual report and other financial information
- Investment in research and development

Appendix 3
Gap Analysis (for an organ-transplant clinic)

Selection Criterion	Vendor 1	Vendor 2	Vendor 3	Vendor 4	Vendor 5
Sites Implemented					
The ability to schedule based on patient-specific, dynamic information, including lab tests, to process the patients more effectively.	X	X	No	X	Future plan.
A tickler list that alerts the staff regarding what laboratory studies are ordered for a specific time frame.	X	X	X	X	X
An interface to receive a select set of laboratory studies from the lab information system.	X	X	X	X	X
The ability to enter discrete lab data that were not completed at a Geisinger lab along with Geisinger laboratory values in chronological order, for comparison to previous lab results.	X	X	Future plan, no date set.	X	X
A field that includes the name of the lab (internal or external) where the test was completed, for comparing results over time.	X	X	X	X	X
The ability to track pre-transplant patients and their workup progress so that the staff can easily determine what has been done and what is required.	X	X	X	X	X
The ability to track patient and living donor information from the time of transplant throughout the post transplant period with only a few keystrokes.	X	X	? Future plan; 1st quarter 2004.	X	X
The ability to connect the donor information to the transplant recipient for quick reference when required.	X	X	X	X	X
Quick reference to the last height, weight, creatinine, and current medications.	X	X	X	X	X
A field to store addresses and phone numbers of pertinent medical providers, such as primary care provider and referring physician.	X	X	X	X	X
The ability to track the patient's dialysis unit address, phone number, and hours of operation to provide ongoing communication with the facility and determine referral patterns.	X	X	X	X	X

Continued

Selection Criterion	Vendor 1	Vendor 2	Vendor 3	Vendor 4	Vendor 5
An electronic medication list, which includes start and stop dates, to record the patient's current medications, the history of previous medications, and future medications.	X	X	X	X	X
A medication list, consisting of pull down menus, that can be maintained by department, which includes the specific adult and pediatric dosages for each medication.	X	X	X	X	X
The ability to update pull down menus with new information as needed.			X	X	X
A quick and easy way to gather information on medicines used to treat transplant rejection episodes.	X	X	No	X	X
The ability to record both inpatient and outpatient results in one location.	X	X	X	X	X
A patient-specific flow sheet, as well as methods to track multiple patients, that includes laboratory results, current medications, biopsy results, rejection treatments, diagnosis, infections, patient status, hospitalizations, and history of cancers for reference and to assist with treatment.	X	X	Need to create report.	X	X
Track multiple transplants (and failed transplants) for the same patient.	X	X	X	X	X
Track patients who receive islet cells with store all pertinent transplant information in one database.	X	?	Future plan, not date set.	X	?
Calculate age in years for adult patients and in days, weeks, and months for pediatric patients.	X	Calculates in tenths (i.e. 6 months = 0.5).	No	After demo we were told that the function was added.	No
Calculation of transplant organ(s) age in years, days, weeks, and months for reporting and research.	X	Not visible on screen. Can set up report.	X	X	X
The ability to track non-US citizens and receive an alert when the number of transplants are near the quota allowed, for compliance with regulatory requirements.	Can set up report to track. No alert.	Can set up report to track. No alert.	Can set up report to track. No alert.	Can set up report to track. No alert.	Can set up report to track. No alert.

Selection Criterion	Vendor 1	Vendor 2	Vendor 3	Vendor 4	Vendor 5
A searchable field to assign or reassign a transplant coordinator to a specific patient and the ability for the transplant coordinator to create the list of their patients or all patients.	X	X	X	X	X
User friendly, customizable pull-down menus for intuitive entry of data.	X	X	X	X	X
The option to sort data fields in both ascending and descending order.	X	No	X	X	X
Customized lists are automatically maintained as application upgrades are applied (to ensure continuity of user defined data).	X	X	X	X	X
Deactivate items from lists but maintain the items for historical purposes.	X	X	X	X	X
The ability to install the application on multiple workstations throughout inpatient and outpatient sites for quick access to transplant information.	X	X	X	X	X
Review a patient's record simultaneously at multiple workstations, allowing one user write access and others read-only access.	Second user will get a message that someone updated the record since it was opened.	Second user will get a message that someone updated the record since it was opened.	Not sure.	No	X
Expand the software to other transplant procedures, such as liver and heart transplants.	X	X	Future plan for pancreas & liver. No plan for heart and lung. X	X	X
Segregate data according to transplant organ, along with sharing data across multiple transplants when needed.	X	X	X	X	X
Patient identification visible on the screen to ensure that staff document on the correct patient.	X	X	X	X	X
The ability to merge and unmerge data that is entered incorrectly or entered on the wrong patient.	Can merge records but can not unmerge.	No	No	The vendor can complete the merge upon request.	No

Continued

Selection Criterion	Vendor 1	Vendor 2	Vendor 3	Vendor 4	Vendor 5
An audit trail to track access and modifications to ensure HIPAA compliance.	Edit-only audit trail. (does not record read-only use.)	Edit-only audit trail. (does not record read-only use.)	Edit-only audit trail. (does not record read-only use.)	X	Edit-only audit trail. (does not record read-only use.)
Send data using a wireless solution, such as a tablet PC, to allow the staff to document during the patient appointment.	Future plan. No date set.	Future plan. No date set.	No	No	Wireless PC only.
Track UNOS required data fields and revise data fields when UNOS revises their data requirements.	X	X	Not sure.	X (Extra cost.)	X
Auto-populate data fields on UNOS forms to decrease redundant documentation and save time.	X	X	No	X (except malignancy and living donor)	X
Transplant candidate registration form	X	No	No	X	X
Kidney transplant registration form	X	No	No	X	X
Kidney/Pancreas transplant registration form	X	No	No	X	X
Pancreas transplant registration form	X	No	No	X	X
Kidney transplant recipient form	X	X	No	X	X
Pancreas transplant recipient follow-up	X	X	No	X	X
Kidney/Pancreas transplant recipient follow-up	X	X	No	X	X
Immuno follow-up	X	X	No	X	X
Living donor registration form	No. (will implement in future.)	No	No	No	X
Living donor follow-up	No. (will implement in future.)	No	No	No	X
Post-Transplant Malingnacies	No. (will implement in future.)	No	No	No	X
Includes a checkbox for malignancies	X	X	Future plan.	X	X
If yes is checked for malignancies, system prompts for all UNOS fields for malignancies	Most fields. Will add all fields when UNOS form is auto-populated.	Most fields. Will add all fields when UNOS form is auto-populated.	Future plan.	Most fields.	X
Track living donor information for UNOS reporting.	X	X	X	X	X
Download all active transplant data from Excel spreadsheet to ensure an inclusive transplant database.	X	X	X	X	X

Appendix 4

		Priority Setting Criteria			
Rank	Project	Value	Need	Strategy	Precedence
1	Clinical Respository				
2	Physician Workstation Tools				
3	Ambulatory Practice System Clinical Data Flow Re-engineering				
4	Laboratory Replacement Systems				
5	Systems				
6	Clinical Order Communications Patient Care Automation				
7	Devices				
.					
.					
.					
.					
.					
.					
.					
n	*Last Project*				

Key: High | Medium | Low

Priority Setting Criteria

1. **Value:** The relationship of cost and benefits.

Significant
Direct Benefits
Few Direct
Benefits

2. **Need:** The importance of the project to the user, strong sponsorship, absence of automation and/or aging information systems no longer providing adequate support.
High = Required
Medium = Important
Low = Beneficial, but
Optional

3. **Supports Strategy:**
A. Help grow the business.
B. Reduce cost of services.
C. Enhance customer satisfaction.
D. Enable patient flow across the organization.
E. Enhance managed care.
F. Improve and measure quality of care.

4. Precedence:
High = Required for most new applications to be successful
Medium = Required for some new applications to be successful
Low = Required for a few new applications to be successful

Appendix 5
Site Characteristics Questionnaire

1. Complete clinic statistics spreadsheet listing:
   a. Clinic hours
   b. Employees and duties
   c. Number of exam rooms (Attach blueprint when possible.)
   d. Number of office visits annually
   e. Number of clinic patients
   f. Site specialties and sub-specialties
   g. Ancillary services
   h. Outreach services and locations
2. Observe each employee's duties:
   a. Check in
   b. Check out
   c. Secretarial support
   d. Nurses
   e. Technicians
   f. Ancillary staff
   g. Mid-level providers (e.g., physician's assistants, CRNPs)
   h. Residents
   i. Physicians
3. List the following for each ancillary area:
   a. Patient-care provided
   b. Duties of all caregivers and support personnel
   c. Document:
      i. Order management
      ii. Patient scheduling
      iii. Review of test results
      iv. Patient billing
4. List processes and procedures related to research activities.
5. Document appointment scheduling processes:
   a. Appointment types
   b. Combined appointments (lab, ancillary, physician)
   c. Special procedures
   d. No-show policies and procedures
6. Document patient messaging flow:
   a. Nurse triage protocols
   b. Medication refill protocols

7. Patient care processes:
   a. Messaging
   b. Check in
   c. Check out
   d. Nursing
      i. Where are vitals taken and documented?
      ii. Where are immunizations administered?
   e. Test ordering
   f. Referral ordering
8. Observe and document interactions with other clinical areas and departments.
9. Observe and document interactions with ancillaries.
10. Collect examples of and document the use of:
    a. Patient instructions
    b. Documentation forms
    c. Order sheets
    d. Billing sheets
    e. Flowcharts
    f. Questionnaires
    g. Clinical drawings
11. Document paper medical record use to support patient care and messaging.

Appendix 6
Low Back Pain

The sixteen diagnostic criteria for new-onset low-back pain from Richard Deyo. Lower back pain; an update. In: American College of Physicians; 1992; San Diego: American College of Physicians; 1992. Tape 1-J.

1. Personal history of cancer (except skin)
2. Unexplained weight loss
3. Fever
4. Long-term steroid use
5. Urinary retention
6. Saddle anesthesia
7. Fecal incontinence
8. Trauma
9. Sciatica
10. Bone pain
11. Spine tender to percussion
12. Breast abnormalities (consistent with cancer)
13. Ipsilateral straight-leg raising
14. Crossed straight-leg raising
15. Ankle dorsiflexion weakness
16. Great toe extensor weakness

Appendix 7

#	Scenarios	Expected Results	Tester Initials	Date Tested	GWV Service Area	GHS Employed User	GHS Non-employed User Respected	Ambulatory EC Classic Verified	Ambulatory EC Verified	Hyper Verified	Space Verified	EpicWeb Verified	EMR Link Verified	Pass/Fail	Comments
1	Cadence/Prelude: Make changes to Northern Region Patient's demographic information and verify changes appear correctly in Hyperspace demographics and SnapShot reports: Contact Information • Permanent Comments • Address • Phone Numbers • DOB • Sex • Social Security Number • Reference/Emergency Contact Changes	1. Log into Hyperspace with all Phase 1 ID for GMC provider. 2. Highlight patient on patient list. 3. Open patient's chart. 4. Review Demographics activity. (Appropriate fields should not be editable.) 5. Verify changes on face sheet reports (from patient lists and patient summary activity). 6. Log into Classic with same ID. 7. Identify patient. 8. Review demographics activity. Verify that only appropriate fields are visible and that data is appropriate. 9. MU 13 Specific—Demographics/Prelude lock should be in place when simultaneously accessing information. User name should display in message.													
2	Follow scenario used in # 1.	1. Log into Hyperspace with all Phase 1 ID for GMC employee (not provider) 2. Highlight patient on patient list 3. Open patient's chart. 4. Review Demographics activity. (Appropriate fields should not be editable.) 5. Verify changes on face sheet reports (from patient lists and patient summary activity). 6. Log into Classic with same ID. 7. Identify patient. 8. Review demographics activity. Verify that only appropriate fields are visible and that data is appropriate.													

Continued

3	Follow scenario used in # 1.	1. Repeat above steps for a GWV employed provider.
4	Follow scenario used in # 1.	1. Repeat above steps for a GWV employee whose is not a provider.
5	Follow scenario used in # 1.	1. Log into Hyperspace with all Phase 1 ID for GWV non-employed provider. 2. Should be stopped, when trying to identify patient, since a Northern Region patient. 3. Log into Classic with same ID. 4. Should be stopped, when trying to identify patient, since a northern region patient.
6	Cadence/Prelude: Make changes to GWV Service Area Region. Access patient's demographic information and verify that changes appear correctly in Hyperspace demographics and SnapShot reports: Contact Information • Permanent Comments • Address • Phone Numbers • DOB • Gender • Social Security Number	1. Log into Hyperspace with all Phase 1 ID for GMC provider. 2. Highlight patient on patient list 3. Open patient's chart. 4. Review Demographics activity. Appropriate fields should not be editable. 5. Verify changes on face sheet reports (from patient lists and patient summary activity). 6. Log into Classic with same ID. 7. Identify patient. 8. Review demographics activity. Verify that only appropriate fields are viewable and that data appropriate.
7	Follow scenario used in # 6.	1. Repeat above steps for a non-provider GMC employee.
8	Follow scenario used in # 6.	1. Repeat above steps for a GWV employee provider.
9	Follow scenario used in # 6.	1. Repeat above steps for a GWV employee who is not a provider.
10	Follow scenario used in # 6.	1. Repeat above steps for a non-employed GWV provider.

#	Scenarios	Expected Results	Tester Initials	Date Tested	GWV Service Area	GHS Employed User Respected	GHS Non-employed User Verified	Ambulatory EC Classic Verified	Ambulatory EC Verified	Hyper Verified	Space Verified	EpicWeb Verified	EMR Link Verified	Pass/Fail	Comments
11	Enter test results (Enter/Edit Results) in Classic and verify each appears correctly in Hyperspace Chart Review for an inpatient.	1. Enter Lab Orders in Classic. 2. Enter results in Classic. 3. Log into Hyperspace. 4. Identify inpatient by location (ward). 5. Verify New Results flag. 6. Select New Results flag (opens results review). 7. Verify that results are viewable in Hyperspace. 8. Set Date/Time stamp. 9. Open Chart Review activity. 10. Verify results on appropriate tab (e.g., lab). 11. Exit Hyperspace.													
12	Edit test results (Enter/Edit Results) in Classic and verify that each appears correctly in the Hyperspace Chart Review Summary for an inpatient.	1. Log into Classic. 2. Edit a result on the same patient according to the above scenario. 3. Log onto Hyperspace. 4. Identify patient on system list for admitted location 5. Verify that New Result flag responds to the edit mode in Classic. 6. Select New Results flag (opens results review). 7. Verify that results are viewable in Hyperspace. 8. Set Date/Time stamp. 9. Open Chart Review activity. 10. Verify results on appropriate tab (lab). 11. Close patient's chart.													

Continued

| 13 | **Cadence user: Insurance Verification. If Primary ins is changed, should be reflected in Hyperspace.** | 1. Log into Hyperspace. 2. Add patient to My List from system list. 3. Highlight patient. 4. View face sheet at bottom for listed insurances. 5. Open patient chart. 6. Select Patient summary activity. 7. View Face Sheet Report for listed insurances. 8. View header for change of insurance. 9. Secure. 10. Verify in Classic that an insurance is listed. 11. Secure. |
| 14 | **Cadence** user: move coverage information to Non-effective coverage. (Use patient in above scenario.) If insurance is moved to non-effective, no coverage should be reflected. | 1. Move coverage information to Non-Effective Coverage. 2. Log into Hyperspace. 3. Highlight patient on My List. 4. View face sheet at bottom for changes. 5. Open patient chart. 6. Select patient summary activity. 7. View face sheet report for the changes made. 8. View Hyperspace header to verify insurance removed. 9. Secure. 10. Verify in Classic that an insurance is listed. 11. Secure. 12. Via Cadence, move coverage information to Non-Effective Coverage. 13. No payor should be listed under Coverage. Information in yellow header as well as within encounter, Primary Ins now reflects "No Coverage". 14. Add coverage in Cadence. 15. Verify in Classic that coverage is reflected yellow header and within encounter. |

#	Scenarios	Expected Results	Tester Initials	Date Tested	GWV Service Area	GHS Employed User	GHS Non-employed User Respected	Ambulatory EC Classic Verified	Ambulatory EC Verified	Hyper Verified	Space Verified	EpicWeb Verified	EMR Link Verified	Pass/Fail	Comments
15	**Cadence** user: enter new coverage (use patient in above scenario) and invoke MSP form.	1. Enter new coverage in Cadence. 2. Log into Hyperspace. 3. Highlight patient on My List. 4. View face sheet at bottom for changes. Print group 49000 should no longer show the 'MSP form' (MU 15). 5. Open patient chart. 6. Select patient summary activity. 7. View face sheet report for the changes made. 8. Verify in Classic that coverage is reflected in yellow header and within encounter.													
16	**Cadence/Prelude** County Field Added to Patient Demographics: We've added a new county field to the Patient Demographics window and rearranged a few other fields on the window to accommodate the new field. We've added a new item to the EPT database (item) 75-COUNTY OF RESIDENCE) where your facility can build a category list for use with the new field. Enter/Edit County field on patient in	1. Log into Hyperspace. 2. Open patient chart. 3. Access Demographics activity. 4. Verify that the correct county displays.													
24	**Cadence** scheduler should not be able to access any inpatient departments for scheduling.	1. Log into Cadence. 2. Change dept to BP2. 3. Select appointment entry. 4. Identify patient. 5. Attempt to schedule in inpatient department. 6. Should not be able to schedule patient.													

25	Roster columns display as column option in Hyperspace patient list. Use d ^E>PAF>to edit column list.	1. View system roster from Classic.
		2. Exit Classic.
		3. Log into inpatient with Hyperspace User ID.
		4. Select shared patient list.
		5. Highlight list. Name and MRN will display.
		6. Right click on the list.
		7. Should not be able to change properties or delete list.
		8. (If you log in with your own IT security, security access may allow you to delete the list. If so, STOP, because this deletes from the entire database.)
26	**Cadence** user: Referral testing	1. Order referral in Classic
		2. On order detail, change the referred-by provider's address
		3. Set expiration date for > 6 months.
		4. Verify in Cadence that the changed address is reflected in POS.
		5. Verify that the expiration date defaults in for 6 months.
27	**Cadence** user: Change Permanent comments in Classic and verify on Demographic Change Report (Cad) that change is reflected.	1. Log into Classic
		2. ID patient.
		3. Access Permanent Comments field and enter data.
		4. Accept screen.
		5. Cadence user log into Demographic Change Report and verify the change.
		6. Log into Hyperspace
		7. ID patient
		8. Verfiy Permanent Comment change and view only.
28	**XP PC Specific (Tech Team Info for MU 15):** When timeout feature is set for workstation or role: 1) Verify ability to log back into application without significant delay and 2) Make sure that activities are viewable in bottom toolbar.	

Appendix 8
EHR User Security Policy/Process

1 General Statement of Policy

The purpose of this procedure is to provide a structured process for user security in all Epic environments at the Geisinger Health System.

* **Scope**

This policy applies to any additions, changes and deletions to EHR user security as well as ID and Password Standards and Security Reports. This policy does not include EHR security classifications.

ENVIRONMENT ACCESS:

* **In order for users to have access to the different EHR environments, they must have the following roles or the following guidelines must be met:**
  * **Release Environment**
    * Test new releases and interfaces, and work on related development.
    * Work on changes to the system that aren't ready for the play or production environments.
  * **Training Environment**
    * Work on training set up.
    * Generic User IDs have been developed for trainees.
  * **Play Environment**
    * Review new functionality.
    * Prepare information that will be used in the production environment.
    * "Play" to keep newly learned skills up to date.
  * **Production Environment**
    * Perform their job duties.
    * Support the EHR system. This includes Help Desk staff, EHR technical staff and EHR team members.
* **Access to an environment will only be given after the following requirements have been met:**
  * Person understands the implications of the environment (for example, that the release environment has interfaces running).
  * Person has received the appropriate training.
  * Person has signed the appropriate Confidentiality Statements. (Forms are sent via inter-office mail to the Administrative Director of Security at 17-00.)

- Person receives access to each environment based on a "Need to Know" basis. For example, if a user is a nurse in one site/department and acts as a receptionist in another site/department, the proper security classifications and departments need to be considered. Written authorization must be obtained to grant a user access.
- **Access to a registration-system department and/or center will follow these guidelines:**
  - The department/center site coordinator must approve all end users' security classifications and fill out the appropriate forms.
  - Access to all other departments will be set to "No Access" or "Inquiry-Only Access".
  - Users will not be given update security into a department or center that has not been authorized.
- **Registration-system Inquiry-Only access will follow these guidelines:**
  - Inquiry Only security classifications will not have any update functions—including interactive reports.
  - Users can be given Inquiry-Only security to any department.

USER ACCESS GUIDELINES:

- User security requests will be handled by filling out the appropriate EHR User Security Request Form on the EHR Web Page.
- **All security requests must be completed and approved by the Site Coordinator/ Operations Manager.**
- **In order to add, delete or change user access in the User Master file, a request is required.**
- **Access is only given to valid users, meaning the user must have a legal name. Generic users are NOT allowed (e.g., Test, Provider). The only variation to this rule is the generic nurse users that only have the ability to view the registration-system Arrival List.**
- **New Implementations**: A security request form is filled out by the Site Coordinator/Operation Manager containing all users working at the site. This form is filled out using the EHR Web page and forwarded automatically to the appropriate e-mail Regional mailbox. Each user will be set up in the system by the Regional Team security designee and receive a sealed envelope marked "CONFIDENTIAL" containing their user ID and password, along with password instructions. **The Site Coordinator/Operations Manager/Regional Team may hand out the envelopes after the user has been trained.**
- New users will be prompted at first logon to change their password.
- **After a site is implemented:** If access is needed for new users an electronic request form using the EHR Web page will be filled out by the Site Coordinator/ Operations Manager and automatically sent to the appropriate e-mail Regional mailbox for the North Central Region.
  - New users will be given access to the EHR via a secure e-mail message or through a confidential, sealed interoffice envelope sent directly to the user containing their user ID and password.
  - New users will be prompted at first logon to change their password.
- **Transferring to other sites/departments:** The Site Coordinator/Operations Manager is responsible for completing the required security request documentation in order for a user to have access to a transferring department/site. The site/department that

the user is transferring to is responsible for the security request. This rule also applies to users covering at sites on a temporary basis.

2 Terminations, Transfers and Extended Leaves

TERMINATIONS: leaving the system completely

All terminations will be handled through the IT Epic Team. **Regional personnel will page one of the IT Security Administrators to deactivate the terminated employee. The IT Security Administrators will have an assigned member of the EHR Team logs each step that they take to assure that the termination has been properly addressed.**

The Registration-system EHR Security Administrator will be notified for the reassignment of schedules and other Registration-system issues. The EHR Security Administrator will be notified for the EHR. All changes and communication will be documented on a spreadsheet and maintained by the Epic Program Director.

1) The registration-system EHR Security Administrator will work closely with the site to assure the reassignment of provider schedules. Operations will be responsible for the reassignment of the schedule(s) and Wait List entries.

2) If the terminated employee is a provider, the EHR team will be notified as to who the covering provider should be for the terminated employee with respect to his or her existing In-Basket. This verbal statement will be followed by an e-mail from the covering provider (or their supervising physician) that they accept responsibility as the covering provider and that the EHR team should proceed in forwarding messages from the In-Basket and that he/she is now resuming responsibility for those messages. The effective date and time should be included in this e-mail message. If the covering provider handling future In-Basket messages is different than the provider accepting responsibility for the existing In-Basket messages, the EHR Security Administrator will need to be notified of this information. An e-mail would need to be received from both providers (or their supervising physician) indicating their acceptance of the responsibility.

3) After the above e-mail is received, the EHR Security Administrator will terminate the password of the terminated provider and his/her In-Basket access.

4) After forwarding the In-Basket messages to the covering provider, IT personnel should not "done" the messages from the terminated provider's In-Basket. The messages will remain in that In-Basket.

5) If the terminated provider has any co-signs in his/her In-Basket, the EHR Security Administrator will print the co-signs and fax them to the covering provider. The covering provider will sign off on the co-signs and fax the signed documents back to the EHR Security Administrator. The EHR Security Administrator will scan the co-signs into a co-sign encounter. (Co-signs can not be forwarded from the In-Basket.)

The above steps are also applicable for nursing, front and back office personnel.

6) The EHR Security Administrator will contact the EHR Sr. Systems Analyst if the terminated provider is a transcription/Chart Script user. This information will also be logged on the spreadsheet. The EHR Sr. Systems Analyst will deactivate this functionality and notify transcription.

7) A spreadsheet will be maintained as to terminated employee, communications related to termination, and all messages forwarded, dated and timed. This should

be printed and signed by the two IT employees who accessed the system, effected the changes, and logged them. After all terminated providers/users have had their In-Baskets addressed, the EHR Security Administrator will contact the EHR Program Director and provide him/her with the spreadsheet. The Technical Program Director will run a report from the back end that logs all the activities performed by the terminated provider/user. The Technical Program Director will provide the EHR Program Director with the copy of the report. The EHR Program Director will review the spreadsheet and the report for accuracy.

Terminations for users other than providers
In the User master file:

- Mark the user as "Inactive".
- Remove the user from any In-Basket Classifications.
- At the Mail System prompt; enter NO MAIL.
- Remove all Departments/Centers.
- Remove Prelude Security and EPI Security.
- Soft-delete the user from the system using the (UN)DELETE option.

Termination for providers
In the User master file:

- Mark the user as "Inactive".
- Remove the user from any In-Basket classifications.
- At the Mail System prompt; enter NO MAIL.
- Remove all Departments/Centers.
- Remove Prelude Security and EPI Security.
- Soft-delete the user from the system using the (UN)DELETE option.

In the Provider master file:

- At the ALSO TO PROVIDER prompt; enter NO.
- Set the Out of Office prompt on the GUI side as well as in the provider master file.
- Remove the department, blocks and messages once all schedules are reassigned and Wait List entries are resolved.
- Remove all Visit-Type modifiers and messages.
- Enter NO in the Out of Office section in the field titled "Receive In-Basket Messages".

In template processing, place a hold on all remaining schedules and set the release date and the date of termination. The Referral master file as well as CDIP will be updated with the appropriate information.

- The EHR Security Administrators will review the Human Resources report on a biweekly basis and make the necessary additions/changes/deletions in the system. *The Site Coordinator/Operation Manager in the appropriate region will be notified of any terminations not reported by the EHR WebPage to ensure that proper documentation will follow.*

USER IDS AND PASSWORDS:

- **User IDs**
  - **All provider IDs in the Eastern, Western, and North Central Region** are set up identically to their CDIP/provider number.

- **All other users in the Eastern, Western, and North Central Region** are set up with a numeric-alpha combination user ID with a minimum of 3 characters per User ID.
- **User IDs may not be reused by a different individual.**
- **Passwords**
  - All users are initially assigned a generic password and will be required, via a system-prompt at first logon, to change it.
  - Passwords must be alphanumeric, at least five characters in length, beginning with an alpha character.
  - The system will prompt the user every 180 days to change their password.
  - Passwords can never be reused.
  - *If a user forgets his/her password, the security administrator will reset and expire the user's new generic password in the system. The user will be notified by a "marked private" e-mail message. In urgent circumstances the user can be notified over the telephone, but a particular field in the User Master file, known only to the user, must be verified.*
  - **A new field, Mother's Maiden Name, in the User Masterfile will be required to ensure proper user security verification. This field will be verified by an EHR Security Administrator if a password needs to be reset or the user is inactivated due to "x" number of Failed Logon Attempts.**

CONFIDENTIALITY FORMS:

During the implementation process, the Regional Teams will be responsible for distributing the confidentiality statements. The Site Coordinator/Ops Manager will be responsible for having each user sign the forms.

- New Hires will be required to understand and sign the Human Resources Patient Confidentiality Statement (one time only, filed in Human Resources).
- All EHR users will be required to understand and sign the PASSWORD AUTHORIZATION AGREEMENT. (The original will remain at the site. A copy will be sent to the Administrative Director of Security for GEISINGER at 17-00.)
- All Epic providers will be required to understand and sign the ELECTRONIC SIGNATURE AUTHORIZATION AGREEMENT TO PARTICIPATE (The original will remain at the site. A copy will be sent to the Administrative Director of Security for GEISINGER at 17-00.)
- All EHR and Regional Team members are required to understand and sign the PASSWORD AUTHORIZATION AGREEMENT, the ELECTRONIC SIGNATURE AUTHORIZATION AGREEMENT TO PARTICIPATE and the yearly PATIENT CONFIDENTIALTY STATEMENT administered by the Information Technology department.

SECURITY REPORTS:

- **Failed Logon Attempts**
  - Users will appear on this report after they've failed to logon to the system correctly, regardless on the number of failed attempts.
  - Users will be "inactivated" from the EHR after five (5) consecutive failed logon attempts. Users can call the HelpDesk to be activated. Via phone, the HelpDesk will verify the Mother's Maiden Name field with the user.

- Documentation from the user and the Regional Security Administrator will be required and kept on file for any user with more than 11 failed attempts.
- The Regional Teams will notify users via e-mail, phone or a Staff Message if they've failed to logon correctly after seven attempts.
- The report runs each night at 10:00 P.M. and is sent via e-mail to the EHR Team-leaders, EHR Security Administrators, Regional Teams and Administrative Director of Security.
- **Monthly Regional Audit Report**
  - The user's name, security classifications, service areas, department and center, as well as the Regional Team member that made the change, will appear on the report.
  - This report was developed for tracking purposes.
- **Quarterly Site Report**
  - This report will be distributed to the Site Coordinator/Manager on a quarterly basis for review.
  - The report contains a listing of employees, their titles (if applicable), and security classifications by center or department.
  - The Site Coordinator/Operations Manager will review and respond to the Regional Team with any changes to the list, including terminations and transfers.

SECURITY AUDITS:

- Random security audits by the EHR Security Administrators will be conducted to monitor compliance based on the EHR Security Protocol.
- Audits from outside of GEISINGER are also a possibility.
- Electronic documentation for each security transaction to the User Master file is required.

IDS AND PASSWORDS FOR REGIONAL AND CORE TEAM MEMBERS:

Each EHR Team and Regional Team member is given provider-type EHR access to enable them to research production problems. **Each ID begins with the user name, followed by the title, "system support".**

- *EHR Team and Regional Team members have two User IDs and Passwords in the production environment.*
- *One for troubleshooting (provider access)*
  - *One for system master file access*
  - *If a member of the EHR Team or Regional Team needs to work in a different capacity at a live site, a separate User ID and Password will be set up in the system.*
- *The appropriate security documentation must be completed and kept on file*
- After access is no longer needed, the user must be inactivated until future use. The same ID and password can be reused as long as the appropriate documentation is completed and kept on file.

Appendix 9

Geisinger Health System	Project Topic:		Responsibilities Document EpicCare Specialty Implementations
Issue	Clinic/Ops Responsibility	IT Responsibility	Notes
General Considerations	Time requirement estimates are just that. The actual time spent on a particular task or issue will vary depending on the clinic size, degree of complexity of work-flows, level of standardization within the clinic, and extent of familiarity with clinic processes. Time estimates do not include the time required to communicate the issues discussed to other clinic staff and it should be assumed that this will be needed to some extent for most aspects of the implementation. When an individual becomes part of a team working on any aspect of the implementation, they are responsible for keeping informed about issues covered at meetings, even when they are unable to attend. Assignment deadlines will not be changed to accommodate for a missed meeting.		Geisinger Health System meeting rules will be applied to the meetings, e.g., agendas, meeting minutes, etc. **Discussion Points:** Who is responsible for making sure residents/interns are present for training, etc? Is this Medical Education or the Clinic? • *7/10/01 Clinic responsibility with Medical Education as second contact.* Who should be the point of contact for any resident-related issues? • *7/10/01 Lead physician for the Department.*
Time line	Support of, negotiation of, and communication of timeline. Provide input as to what will need to go live along with clinic or department (what ancillary services, etc.) Provide a commitment to procedural changes to accommodate automation. **Estimated Time Requirement:** **2 hr meeting for timeline presentation, and discussion.**	Develops timeline for clinic/department. Communicates when implementation is complete. Provide information about how to obtain new requests once implementation is over. Meet with Sr. VPs to discuss timeline, approach, expectations, responsibilities. Development of a detailed implementation plan.	The details of the clinic timeline will be shared and mutually agreed upon within the framework of the system implementation time line. The scope of what will be going live will be clearly defined at the outset of the process. The time line date for implementation cannot be changed without agreement from the Chief Medical Information Officer and either the Assistant Chief Medical Officer for Medicine or Surgery. An example of a valid reason for changing the time line could include significant, unexpected changes in staffing.

Continued

Geisinger Health System	Project Topic:		Responsibilities Document EpicCare Specialty Implementations
Issue	Clinic/Ops Responsibility	IT Responsibility	Notes
			Assumptions: Post-implementation IT support is separate from implementation. Implementation is considered completed the 4th week after shadowing for Phases 4/5 has ended. Clinic sites will go live with the current EHR functionality. Advanced Charting Tools training sessions are held monthly. Registration for these classes is available through the EHR Info Web page. It will be the clinic's responsibility to have an individual attend a session typically within 6–8 weeks after implementation.
Modified Phase 3 Roll-out	Respond to Modified Phase 3 Team Leader's email requesting number of exam and procedure rooms. Respond to the questionnaire. Determine if devices need to be placed in the exam rooms for this phase. Assure that personnel including residents are scheduled and attend the training sessions (including the blocking of provider schedules). **(1 hr, one time)** Define the department procedure for additional dictation needs. Assure that the staff has an understanding of EHR Results Review functionality. Assign a key resource who will take primary responsibility for ensuring that folks are using MP3, act as the key contact with IT,	Provide additional devices if necessary. Provide training. Provide the questionnaire and the transcription document types that will be used by each department. Provide recommended workflows. Provide shadowing support. Clean up phrase file. Analyze and build user classes and pools.	A standardized workflow for transcription will be developed to address the distribution of mailings and cc's. **Assumptions:** The standard transcription-to-EHR workflows and filing process will be followed. There will be no customization of this process. If an area requests devices for the exam rooms, the implementation will proceed even if Facilities cannot accommodate the timeline for renovations.

Continued

and act as a subject matter expert within their clinic. Write Out of Office Policy, communicate to staff **(2 hrs, one time)**
Develop understanding of clinic message and phone call flow, including transcriptions.
Identify individuals who will participate in pool and class development. **(4 hrs, one time)**
Assist in pool and class analysis and development. **(2 hrs, one time)**

Assumption:
System Access Committee may need to have input into this process.

Review of Scheduling-System Practices	Meet with IT representatives to review current scheduling system practices and templates. Review to include Danville clinics as well as Geisinger Outreach sites.	Completion of the scheduling-system tool-kit to identify scheduling issues and practices which will need to be addressed prior to EHR implementation.
Pre-Kick-Off	Schedule meeting and appropriate attendees (minimum: Vice President, Administrative Provider, Operations Manager). Schedule meeting location that meets needs outlined by IT. Process by which decisions will be made will be defined (consensus in clinic vs. individual w/ primary responsibility vs. other). Identify responsible individuals who will be advocates for the project (Super users, Ops people). The identified personnel must be available for the go-live of all phases. Oversight meetings with the lead personnel will be held ad hoc. Identify a lead physician for the implementation who actively pursues and achieves buy-in from their peers. **Estimated Time of Involvement: 4 hrs to schedule meeting, identify project advocates, and communicate roles to these individuals 1–2 hrs for the actual meeting**	Provide Ops with meeting room requirements—if necessary. (e.g., phone line, screen) Review: • High level timeline • Scope of implementation—to include identification of issues such as ancillary areas or niche systems for which analysis shall occur. Analysis is for assessment, and does not mean that all ancillary areas are included in the implementation or interfaces always developed. • Development deadlines • Implementation plan • Type of support needed • Role of control team members • Site responsibilities and tasks

Agenda to include the establishment of ground rules for the implementation.
Discussion Points:
Need to define "Domain Expert/Super Users" and what their role will be.
• *7/10/01 Domain Expert/Super User Document developed by EHR team for Clinic.*
Define how missed deadlines will be addressed.
• *7/10/01 The issues escalation and missed deadlines process will be defined during this Pre-kickoff meeting.*

Geisinger Health System	Project Topic:		Responsibilities Document EpicCare Specialty Implementations
Issue	Clinic/Ops Responsibility	IT Responsibility	Notes
Kick-off Meeting	Scheduling and set up of meeting place that meets list of needs and personnel. Ensure that staff attends the meeting. Senior Leadership attends meeting and communicates the strategic importance of the EHR implementation, outlines expectations, etc. Decision making process will be communicated to the clinic staff. Present EHR impact on Clinic operations and discuss clinic/ops responsibilities including timeline, deadlines, communication process, tasks, personnel identified to participate in Control Team meetings. **Estimated Time of Involvement: 2 hrs for planning and scheduling of meeting 1–2 hrs for meeting**	Provide a list of needs for the Kick-Off meeting room (network port, screen, etc) which the clinic will provide. Provide a list of required attendees. Bring device and projection equipment as needed for demo. Perform demo, outline expectations.	**Discussion Points:** Need to define who will be referred to when using the term "Senior Leadership." • *7/10/01 "Senior Leadership" is defined as the Associate and Vice President for the area service line.*
Process Flow and Redesign	Assistance with evaluation of flow and redesign. **(6 hrs per week for 4 wks)** Walkthroughs. **(1–2 hrs, one time)** Take responsibility for decisions made. Be the "go-to" person for complaints about workflows. Attend training provided by IT. **(4 hrs, one time)** Clinic responsibility to establish and maintain EHR reference manual. Clinic responsibility to update policies and procedures manual for JACHO to include EHR.	Assistance with workflows assessment and redesign. Provide EpicCare training to selected personnel (Super Users and Ops advocates). Set up of Play-Train environment. Walkthroughs. Decide on maximum number of order transmittal set ups. Provide documents for standard workflows.	Workflow assessment will take place with the understanding that there will be a need for redesign and that standardization of practices is one of the goals of this redesign. There will be clear documentation whenever Clinic/ops decides to deviate from the recommended workflow. • *8/8/01: Documentation must be presented to the multidisciplinary feedback team for review and approval.* Following training of selected personnel, ID's and passwords will be given so these people will be able to familiarize themselves with the EHR.

Preference List Development	Provide input to IT. Return Preference Lists to IT in proper format and in mutually agreed upon timeframe. Lists to be approved using method defined in Pre-Kick-Off meeting. **Estimated Time of Involvement: 3 hr/week for person doing the preference list review and development during this phase of implementation.**	Provide Clinic with a list of expectations regarding how preference lists are developed and the timeline associated with development. Analysis with input from Ops. Provide starter set of preference lists in appropriate format for Clinic/Ops to use when developing lists. Have lists evaluated by billing department.	If deadlines are missed, hen site gets an "off the shelf" preference list. Diagnosis list components must be mapped to ICD-9 codes. • *8/8/01: Finalized preference lists will be signed off by all Clinic providers.*
Control Team Meetings	Schedules people and room, including special invitations to outside sources of information (e.g., billing). Lead physician actively pursues and achieves buy in from peers. Take responsibility for decisions made. Be the "go-to" person for complaints and questions about workflows. Review existing Charting Tools to decide which they want available. **(6hrs, one time)** Identify any unique needs of the clinic (e.g., research plans). Responsible to identify and submit items for agenda 3 days prior to meeting. Distribute meeting minutes and communicate the result of decisions made to the clinic staff. **Additional Estimated Time of Involvement: 3 hrs for completion of the other tasks in this section, which includes attendance at 1 hr/week meeting.**	Provide tasks to be completed including explanations of what is needed to complete the task. Develop meeting agenda and distribute one day prior to meeting. Provide minutes from meetings. Coordination of charting tools development. Provide list of existing carting tools for review. Provide list of existing Reasons for Visit/Call for review.	Focus on short-term tasks with deadlines in immediate future. If control team is very large, consider a smaller advisory team to make preliminary decisions. Cancellation of Control Team Meetings to be mutually agreed upon by Clinic and IT. Significant issues that are not time-critical will be addressed by the multidisciptinany feedback team.

Continued

Project Topic:

Responsibilities Document
EHR Specialty Implementations

Issue	Clinic/Ops Responsibility	IT Responsibility	Notes
Charting Tools Development	Assist in identifying charting tools needs and understand use of these tools. Assist in development by providing clinical information (items for lists, sample notes, etc.) as needed. Arrange for appropriate staff to attend Phase 6 training. **Anticipated Time of Involvement: 3 hrs/week**	Make selected charting tools available. Develop new charting tools based on analysis and input from clinic/ops. 3 note templates will be provided for each clinic. Instruct how discrete data can be captured for reporting purposes without need for a Visual Basic forms.	Following Advanced Charting Tools training, the clinic is responsible to develop charting tools following IT process for naming conventions and Smart Set release. Phrases are considered charting tools.
Training	Ensure that prerequisites have been completed: basic microcomputer skills, Results Review/ (Letter Out), Schedule, (No Show), and MP3. Ensure that billing training has occurred with IT input. Schedule Training times and block schedules. Responsible to assure users attend training. **Anticipated Time of Involvement: 1–2 hrs, one time 8 hrs for attendance at training**	Provide Training (phase 4 & 5). Provide Training materials. Provide Clinic with list of training attendees.	Training will include specifics on some of the charting tools selected for the site. Ops manager should attend training.
Transcription	Ensure compliance with workflows.	Educate regarding transcription flows.	**Assumption:** The standard transcription-to-EHR workflows and filing process will be followed. (There will be no customization of this process.)

Billing	Understand billable procedures for their clinic. Knowledge of clinic billing practices, PA, CRNP, resident billing. Serve as liaison between Billing and IT.	Develop, test and implement billing-system mapping for EHR charge document.	Cover this close to the beginning of the process. Schedule a meeting with Billing to discuss implementation plan, identify issues, work towards resolution, pay close attention to multi-specialty clinics.
Outreach	Identify those providers participating in outreach clinics. Work with IT to establish live date for outreach clinics. Clinic is responsible to maintain user phrase files.	Complete the system set up for the outreach clinic department. Perform analysis of the outreach clinic site current set up and workflows. Train workflow for phrase file copying.	**Assumptions:** Outreach clinic support is for Geisinger clinics. Providers working in outreach sites will follow the site's existing order-transmittal flow.
Issues Lists	Maintain familiarity of the contents of the issues list. Review and communicate information to staff. Assume responsibility for operational issues and communication to staff.	Communicate what is appropriate for the issues list. Development of issues list with input from Ops/Clinic.	Needs to include estimated time frame for resolution. Need to distinguish questions from issues. Identify who put the issue on the list.
Communicating the Implementation to Patients	Provide positive communication to the patient community.	Provide pamphlets and other informational material as available.	Operations and IT are responsible to assure EHR implementation has minimal impact on patients.
Communication	Ongoing communication within the department. Ongoing discussions at OIPT. Support current functionality.	Provide a clear understanding of what functionality will be available in the EHR at the time of go-live. Distributes and discusses Frequently Asked Questions document. Communicate EHR go-live dates to Transcription, Medical Records, Billing Lab, Rad.	
Smart Forms	Gain an understanding of when Visual Basic forms will be developed.	Clearly explain the reasons why Visual Basic forms are developed.	No Visual Basic forms will be developed unless recommended by IT. Efforts will be made to find an alternative to these forms whenever possible.

Appendix 10
Abstraction Form

Provider			

PCP:

	Problem List None [ ]		Comments (e.g., CABG 3/95; EF 40% 4/98; Thall Neg 4/98)
	Problem	**ICD-9 Code**	

	Medication Record Including Supplements		None on Record [ ] If Discontinued:
	Medication + Strength	**Sig**	**Reason for discontinuation**
Ex:	*Ranitidine 150 mg*	*1 po BID*	
1			
19			
20			

	Allergies	NKDA _____		
	Agent	**Date noted**	**Reaction**	**Allergy type (i.e. side effect, systemic?)**
1				
2				
3				
4				
5				

	Immunizations	**None on Record** _____		
		Date given	**Date given**	**Date given**
	DT, most recent			
	Influenza, most recent			
	Pneumococcal vaccine, most recent			
	Hepatitis A	#1	#2	
	Hepatitis B	#1	#2	#3
	MMR	#1	#2	
	Rubella			
	Varicella	#1	#2	
	Lymrix	#1	#2	#3
	Other	#1	#2	
	Other	#1	#2	

Appendix 11
Practice-Analysis Checklist

1. Complete clinic statistics spreadsheet listing:
   a. Clinic hours
   b. Employees and duties (e.g., number of physicians, nurses)
   c. Number of exam rooms (attach blueprint diagram when possible)
   d. Number of annual office visits
   e. Number of clinic patients
   f. Site specialties and sub-specialties
   g. Ancillary services
   h. Outreach services and locations
2. Observe each employee's duties:
   a. Check-in
   b. Check-out
   c. Secretarial support
   d. Nurses
   e. Technicians
   f. Ancillary staff
   g. Physician extenders (e.g., physician assistant, CRNP)
   h. Residents
   i. Physicians
3. List ancillary areas and the following for each:
   a. Describe ancillary patient care
   b. Observe technicians and providers duties
   c. Document:
      i. Order receipt
      ii. Patient scheduling
      iii. Result reporting
      iv. Patient billing
4. List research projects, processes and procedures
5. Document patient appointment scheduling process:
   a. Appointment types
   b. Combined appointments (e.g., lab, ancillary, physician)
   c. Special procedures
   d. No-show policies and procedures
6. Document patient messaging flow:
   a. Nurse triage documents, protocols
   b. Medication refill documents, protocols

7. Patient care analysis:
   a. Patient messaging
   b. Patient check-in
   c. Patient check-out
   d. Patient-care workflows
      i. Where vitals are taken and documented
      ii. Where immunizations are administered
   e. Test order workflows
   f. Referral order workflows
8. Observe and document interaction with other clinical areas and departments.
9. Observe and document interaction with ancillaries.
10. Collect examples of and document use:
    a. Patient care forms
    b. Patient care documentation forms
    c. Order sheets
    d. Billing sheets
    e. Flowcharts
    f. Questionnaires
    g. Drawings on which patient data is recorded.
11. Document paper medical record flows during patient care and messaging.

Appendix 12

IS Policy 02.02.01
Subject: Clinical Information System (CIS) Needs and Feasibility Analyses
Effective Date: February 1, 2002

POLICY: The business plan for projects including an electronic information system with potential clinical application (including "freeware" and systems included with the purchase of other items, e.g., monitors) will include an analysis of the business needs, benefits, operational costs, and information system feasibilities of the information system.

PURPOSE: To provide complete, accurate information to decision makers regarding the System-wide information-systems implications of proposed clinical information systems purchases and development.

DEFINITION: *Strategic (or core) clinical-information systems* are systems which GHS has made an integral part of its enterprise-wide, long-term business plan. They extend across the entire Health System, spanning service lines, departments, and sites. Substantial purchase, development, training, and maintenance costs for these systems are included in the ongoing Information Systems budget. (Examples are the EHR systems and the Stentor/IDX image-management system.)

PROCEDURE:
1. The requesting clinical business unit(s)—in consultation with other relevant stakeholders throughout GHS—will document the clinical and business need(s) to be fulfilled by the information system.
2. The EVP, COO and/or EVP, CMO or their designees will confirm that all relevant stakeholders have been included.
3. Information Systems and the requesting clinical business unit(s) together will assess which identified IT needs are supported by existing, strategic systems.
4. Information Systems will estimate when the remaining identified IT need(s) will be supported by a strategic system.
5. If appropriate, Information Systems and the requesting clinical business unit(s) will document due diligence in assessing the market and selecting a potential new clinical-information system.
6. The Information Security office will provide an assessment of the compliance of any proposed clinical information system with GHS information-security standards, HIPAA, and other external regulations. It will estimate the resource costs—to Information Systems and to the clinical business unit(s)—of meeting the relevant standards.

7. Information Systems will estimate purchase costs, implementation costs, maintenance costs, resource availabilities, effects on current projects, and a service-level agreement in consultation with the requesting department(s).
8. The clinical business unit(s) will complete the standard ROI analysis and capital request as supported by Finance and Business Strategy & Development.
9. Business Strategy & Development will confirm the completion of 1–8 and include the information in the relevant business plan.

Responsibility: As above

Document Information
Devised: December, 2001
Revised/Reviewed: January, 2003
Approved: January 15, 2002

APPROVED BY: CISOC, Clinical Operations

Appendix 13
Reference Call Outline
Geisinger Information Services

The focus of the call should be on the success of the implementation and training, the vendor's record for problem response and resolution, enhancement support, overall system satisfaction and the business relationship with the vendor(s).

Vendor: _____

Client: _____

Application: _____

Contact Name: _____

Title and Department: _____

Do you receive any consideration (financial or other) from the vendor for conducting reference calls like this one? _____ Yes _____ No

I. Selection Process

What factors prompted you to purchase the system? What were the organizational drivers? What were your objectives? Have they been achieved?

Which vendors were involved in your final selection group?

_____

What was the project/system budget/price range? _____

How/why was the final vendor selected? _____

What would you do differently if you were to select the system again?

_____

Would you choose this vendor again? Why or why not? _____ Yes _____ No

_____

Was a cost-benefit analysis or any ROI analysis completed? If yes, briefly summarize the findings.

    Increased volume of procedures? _____

    Decreased cost per procedure? _____

    Physician time _____

    Support staff _____

    Room and equipment costs _____

    Software-system cost per procedure? _____

What products/applications are live?

_____

What is planned for future implementation? What is the implementation schedule?

What is the scheduled downtime and unscheduled downtime?

What is the reaction time from the vendor for issue resolution? Examples:

Have you customized the system? If yes, to what degree?

Have you completed an upgrade? What was that process like? Did you have any issues? Was any current functionality removed with the upgrade? Have you upgraded any of your equipment? What brand of equipment do you use? How did you assure that this product will interface with new equipment, perhaps from a different vendor? How are prior customizations dealt with during an upgrade?

What interfaces are in place, required? How are they contracted for and installed? What issues did you encounter in the development of the interfaces?

Do you have a redundant production system? What is your disaster recovery approach?

Do you have an archive strategy? If yes, what is your plan?

Who are the key users of the system (e.g., physicians, nurses)? How do they respond to the system?

What are the principal strengths of the system?

What are the principal weaknesses of the system?

TRAINING AND IMPLEMENTATION

What pre- and post-implementation training was provided by the vendor? How effective was it?

How long was the implementation process? _____

What resources were required from what departments for implementation?

What resources were required from IT for implementation?

What kind of support did your hospital receive from the vendor throughout the implementation, from the planning phase through the post-implementation review?

_____

What was the impact on the departments during the implementation? Afterwards?
     Productivity _____
     Work effort _____
     Morale   _____
How have your staffing patterns changed since the system was installed?

_____

What is considered an adequate training time for a new employee on the system (in hours)?
     Physician   _____
     Nursing   _____
     Clerical   _____
If you could change anything in the system, what would it be?

_____

What specific operational or organizational problems has the system solved?

_____

What specific problems (operational, organizational) has it created?

_____

INFORMATION SYSTEMS
(For Information Systems representatives)

What level of expertise is required for the IT department to support the system?

_____

What system features require special programming?

_____

What are the system security features?

_____

What are the system backup procedures?

_____

What seems to be the most difficult aspect of the system from the IT standpoint?

_____

Was the vendor staff knowledgeable about the system/project? _____
Does the system have a report writer? Who uses it? Is it easy to use?

_____

Rate the performance of the database and associated tools.

_____

Is the system response time acceptable to users?

_____

Did the software and hardware vendors consistently meet your expectations during the implementation? _____

Did the vendors (software/hardware) work in a cooperative manner (i.e., working together to solve problems)?

_____

Describe any other technical issues.

_____

_____

Glossary

Abstracting—entering patient data from a paper medical record into the EHR (e.g., problem lists, medications, medical history)

Academic Detailing—one-on-one or small-group educational outreach to physicians and other clinicians intended to optimize their management of medical conditions and use of healthcare resources

ADT (Admission/Discharge/Transfer)—a system for tracking a patient's hospital admission status from admission through any transfers to discharge

Analyst, Implementation Analyst—one who studies a practice's workflows and information-management needs in order to plan and implement EHR software choices to meet those needs

Authority (Prescribing Authority, Ordering Authority)—an organization's assignment of responsibility for ordering medications or tests to a caregiver type. This assignment is based on the requirements of external regulators and payers and on internal needs for quality of care, workflow standardization, and efficiency

Build, EHR Build—the sum of the configuration choices (regarding, e.g., what functions will be available to which users) made in the course of implementing an EHR

Caregiver types—in the United States these include: attending physicians, fellows, residents, medical students, psychologists, physician assistants (PA), certified registered nurse practitioners (CRNP), clinical nurse specialists (CNS), registered nurses (RN), licensed nurse practitioners (LPN), medical assistants (MA), certified nurse midwifes (CNM), diagnostic technicians, anti-coagulation pharmacists, registered dietitians, clinical office support staff, and non-clinical office support staff

Care Management—a comprehensive program of healthcare services designed to enable patients to achieve maximum well being and independence

Change order—a request, usually from an EHR user, for a change in the EHR system build, e.g., for the addition of a diagnosis that is absent from (or hard to find in) ICD-9

Clinician—any healthcare practitioner (See caregiver types.)

Clinician Domain Expert—see Chapter 9, Clinical Decision Support

Clinical prediction rule—a decision-making tool that uses variables from the history, physical examination, and/or simple diagnostic tests to provide an estimate of the likelihood of a medical or surgical condition

Cognitive load—the amount of information that must be retained in working memory and processed consciously in order to use a system (such as an EHR)

Comprehension—the interpretation of symbols into meaningful information—the final stage of reading (Scanning is the first.)

Customization—used in two overlapping, but distinguishable meanings:
- An optimized implementation involves detailed process analysis and the creation of specialized EHR components like preference lists, order sets, and notes templates for each different clinical business unit. None of this should require changes in the EHR's code.
- While we avoid it wherever possible, optimization sometimes requires software programming changes—performed by our own or the software vendor's programmers.

Demand Management—any of a variety of administrative and clinical services designed to reduce unnecessary use of healthcare services

Domain Expert—see Chapter 9, Clinical Decision Support

e-messaging—This is a secure variant of e-mail in which the message remains on a Web server protected by https (secure hypertext transfer protocol). The recipient reads the message through an encrypted, secure Internet connection, usually after logging into the Web server. (An e-mail notification that a message is available may be sent via unsecured e-mail.)

Effectiveness—whether an intervention (e.g., an active alert or an EHR) works in everyday use

Efficacy—the ability of an intervention (e.g., an active alert or an EHR) to produce specific effects in ideal conditions, that is, in a research setting with highly trained staff who have a specific interest in the intervention

EHR—electronic health record

Environment—see Play Environment and Test Environment

Fault Tolerance—the ability of a system or component to continue normal operation despite the presence of hardware or software faults

Fiscal Year—accounting year (vs. calendar year)

Hard Stop—a software feature that prohibits any further system action until a required prior action (for example, providing data in a field) is completed

Healthcare Informatics—the art and science of fulfilling the clinical-information needs of the various participants in healthcare (i.e., patients, physicians, nurses, other clinicians and caregivers, administrative personnel, researchers, payers, and regulators)

Healthcare Informatician—one who develops, implements, studies, or maintains clinical information systems

IAM (identity and access management)—a security system that enables users to identify themselves and get facilitated access to appropriate software applications and services

ICD Codes—The International Classification of Diseases of the World Health Organization is a billing terminology, which is often pressed into service as a clinical terminology. For clinicians, it is markedly less precise and less usable than is SNOMED (another terminology).

Implementation Analyst—one who studies a practice's workflows and information-management needs in order to plan and implement EHR software choices to meet those needs

Informatician—one who designs, develops, implements, studies or maintains information systems

Institute of Medicine (IOM)—a nonprofit organization chartered in 1970 as a component of the National Academy of Sciences. Its mission is to advance and disseminate scientific knowledge to improve human health; the Institute provides influential white papers concerning healthcare.

Interface—communication channel between computer systems

Just-In-Time Learning—training that occurs just when the learner needs it

Legacy System—a software system so old that it works

Master File—a database file that contains static records used to identify entities such as EHR users, work centers, diagnoses or appointment types

Medical—a term that has historically been used to designate either what is increasingly called healthcare or matters relating to physicians (e.g., medical school)

Medical Informatician—see healthcare informatician

Mid-level Provider—one who provides patient care and orders tests and treatments under a supervisory arrangement with a physician

Navigation—"the ways users make their way from one part of the system to another, including moving from menu to menu, moving within a single screen, moving from screen to screen . . ." (1)

Pattern Matching—the presentation of items in a picklist based on the letters in their names matching exactly the letters typed into an appropriate field. For example, if an EHR user types "amox" into a drug-ordering field, various formulations of amoxicillin will appear in a picklist.

Pend an order—to initiate an order that will not be released for action until an authorized EHR user finalizes it

Play Environment—a non-production version of the EHR that provides the users the opportunity to practice using the EHR with no risk that they will alter real patients' records or otherwise affect the production EHR

Precision Healthcare—provision of evidence-based care to everyone and inappropriate care to no one (2)

Preference List—a short (usually less than 200 items) list of diagnoses, medications, or non-medication orders that the user sees first when she enters a word or phrase into the appropriate search field

Primary-Care Provider—in the United States, a generalist physician, i.e., family practitioner, pediatrician, internist

Project Management—the process of planning and organizing people and other resources to accomplish an objective. (For more information, go to the Project Management Institute at http://www.pmi.org/info/default.asp.)

Provider—one who orders patient tests and treatments; usually a physician or mid-level provider

Readability—Reading is comprised of two stages, scanning and comprehension. Readability is improved by displaying information so that it is either more easily scanned or more easily comprehended (or both). EHR design affects both scanning (e.g., is the abnormal result hidden in a forest of less important data or do color and spacing make it prominent?) and comprehensibility (e.g., are the creatinine results converted to GFR estimates so that renal function can be graphed, to show the decline in function at a glance?).

Root-cause analysis—tracing the causes of a failure from the proximate causes to the primary (root) causes

RVU (Revenue Value Unit)—a measure widely used to compare the productivity of physicians

Scope Creep—the inexorable expansion of a project's goals, usually resulting from a failure to agree on the goals in advance and to keep the project team's work focused on those goals

Screen Shot (or screen capture)—an image of a computer screen's contents at a particular moment. (Screen shots are often useful for illustrating aspects of the EHR's system build.)

Security Token—a small device which authenticates a user for remote sign-in, e.g., a key fob with a number generator synchronized with a server. (When added to a unique user ID and password, a security token provides two-factor authentication.)

Shadow Server—a secondary server running a constantly updated copy of the production application; this server provides a fully functional copy of the application to users when the production server is unavailable. It also allows searches of the application's data without slowing the production server's speed and provides remote access to the application without compromising data security.

Shadowing (Shadow Training)—the provision of trainers wherever and whenever clinicians work, typically beginning at system go-live and lasting two weeks

Shadowing, Shadow Support—user support in which a trainer follows users (unobtrusively) through their normal work routine in order to identify opportunities for just-in-time training, to answer questions, and to minimize frustration; provided wherever and whenever clinicians work, beginning at system go-live and lasting about two weeks

Source system—a separate information system that feeds data into the EHR (e.g., a laboratory information system)

Stakeholder—a party or individual with a natural or organizationally defined role in shaping an agreement or project

Super User—a member of a practice's staff with special interests, training and skills in helping fellow practice members use the EHR effectively

Supervising Provider—a caregiver with the authority and responsibility to finalize orders and other care processes initiated by other caregivers

System Build—the sum of the configuration choices (regarding, e.g., what functions will be available to which users) made in the course of implementing an EHR

Test Environment—a non-production version of the EHR which gives the technical team the opportunity to test the EHR with no risk that they will alter real patients' records or otherwise affect the production EHR

Virtual Feedback Group—a group of physicians who provide (by e-mail) expanded, organization-wide feedback on carefully focused implementation questions from multidisciplinary feedback teams

References

1. Weiss E. Making Computers People-Literate. San Francisco: Jossey-Bass; 1998.
2. Brook R. The cost-quality interface. In: Walker J, editor. Translating Evidence into Practice; Washington, D.C.; 1997.

Index

Health Informatics Series
(formerly Computers in Health Care)

(continued from page ii)

Introduction to Clinical Informatics
P. Degoulet and M. Fieschi

Behavioral Healthcare Informatics
N.A. Dewan, N.M. Lorenzi, R.T. Riley, and S.R. Bhattacharya

Patient Care Information Systems
Successful Design and Implementation
E.L. Drazen, J.B. Metzger, J.L. Ritter, and M.K. Schneider

Evaluation Methods in Biomedical Informatics, Second Edition
C.P. Friedman and J.C. Wyatt

Introduction to Nursing Informatics, Second Edition
K.J. Hannah, M.J. Ball, and M.J.A. Edwards

Strategic Information Management in Hospitals
An Introduction to Hospital Information Systems
R. Haux, A. Winters, E. Ammenwerth, and B. Brigl

Information Retrieval
A Health and Biomedical Perspective, Second Edition
W.R. Hersh

The Nursing Informatics Implementation Guide
E.C. Hunt, S.B. Sproat, and R.R. Kitzmiller

Information Technology for the Practicing Physician
J.M. Kiel

Computerizing Large Integrated Health Networks
The VA Success
R.M. Kolodner

Medical Data Management
A Practical Guide
F. Leiner, W. Gaus, R. Haux, and P. Knaup-Gregori

Consumer Health Informatics
Informing Consumers and Improving Health Care
D. Lewis, G. Eysenbach, R. Kukafka, P.Z. Stavri, and H. Jimison

Organizational Aspects of Health Informatics, Second Edition
Managing Technological Change
N.M. Lorenzi and R.T. Riley

Transforming Health Care Through Information, Second Edition
N.M. Lorenzi, J.S. Ash, J. Einbinder, W. McPhee, and L. Einbinder

Trauma Informatics
K.I. Maull and J.S. Augenstein

Health Informatics Series
(formerly Computers in Health Care)

Consumer Informatics
Applications and Strategies in Cyber Health Care
R. Nelson and M.J. Ball

Public Health Informatics and Information Systems
P.W. O'Carroll, W.A. Yasnoff, M.E. Ward, L.H. Ripp,
and E.L. Martin

Advancing Federal Sector Health Care
A Model for Technology Transfer
P. Ramsaroop, M.J. Ball, D. Beaulieu, and J.V. Douglas

Medical Informatics
Computer Applications in Health Care and Biomedicine, Second Edition
E.H. Shortliffe and L.E. Perreault

Filmless Radiology
E.L. Siegel and R.M. Kolodner

Cancer Informatics
Essential Technologies for Clinical Trials
J.S. Silva, M.J. Ball, C.G. Chute, J.V. Douglas, C.P. Langlotz, J.C. Niland,
and W.L. Scherlis

Clinical Information Systems
A Component-Based Approach
R. Van de Velde and P. Degoulet

Implementing an Electronic Health Record System
J.M. Walker, E.J. Bieber, and F. Richards

Knowledge Coupling
New Premises and New Tools for Medical Care and Education
L.L. Weed

Information Technology Solutions for Healthcare
K. Zieliński, M. Duplaga, and D. Ingram